100 Case Histories for the MRCP

9988

£9-95

For Churchill Livingstone:
Publisher: Laurence Hunter
Project Editor: Dilys Jones
Production Controller: Debra Barrie
Sales Promotion Executive: Marion Pollock

100 Case Histories for the MRCP

Peter S. Sever PhD, FRCP
Professor of Clinical Pharmacology,
St Mary's Hospital Medical School,
Imperial College of Science, Technology
and Medicine, London, UK

Samer Kaddoura BSc, MRCP
Registrar in Medicine and Cardiology,
St Mary's Hospital and Royal Brompton Hospital, London, UK

David J. Spalton FRCP, FRCS, FCOphth
Consultant Ophthalmologist,
St Thomas' Hospital, London, UK

Peter Dorrington Ward MB, BS, MRCP
Consultant Physician,
Manor House Hospital, London, UK

THIRD EDITION

CHURCHILL LIVINGSTONE
EDINBURGH LONDON MADRID MELBOURNE NEW YORK AND TOKYO 1994

CHURCHILL LIVINGSTONE
Medical Division of Longman Group UK Limited

Distributed in the United States of America by Churchill
Livingstone Inc., 650 Avenue of the Americas, New
York, N.Y. 10011, and by associated companies, branches
and representatives throughout the world.

First edition 1976
Second edition 1982
Third edition 1994

ISBN 0-443-04701-4

British Library Cataloguing in Publication Data
A catalogue record for this book is available from the
British Library.

Library of Congress Cataloging in Publication Data

100 case histories for the MRCP / Peter S. Sever . . . [et
al.],—3rd ed.
    p. cm.
    Rev. ed. of: 100 case histories for the MRCP /
David J. Spalton, Peter S. Sever, Peter Dorrington
Ward, 2nd ed. / revised by John Armitstead, Michael
Greenstone. 1982.
    Includes index.
    1. Medicine—Examinations, questions, etc.
2. Medicine—Case studies.   I. Sever, Peter S.
II. Spalton, David J. 100 case histories for the
MRCP.   III. Title: One hundred case histories for the
MRCP.
    [DNLM: 1. Clinical Medicine—examination
questions.   WB 18 Z947 1994]
RC58.S6   1994
616′.0076—dc20
DNLM/DLC
for Library of Congress   93–10622
                                                 CIP

Produced by Longman Singapore Publishers Pte Ltd
Printed in Singapore

Preface

Since the first edition of this book was published in 1976, it has become
established as part of the revision for the majority of candidates taking the
MRCP examination in the UK and has also acquired a large following
amongst those taking similar examinations overseas. The authors have
taken the opportunity in the preparation of this third edition to completely
revise the cases, to include new case material where appropriate and to
emphasise new diagnostic techniques and therapeutic measures. We would
like to thank many of our colleagues who have advised us on the case
material and we hope that this new edition will be thought provoking and
provide assistance to those about to take the MRCP examinations. We also
believe that students not committed to the MRCP examination will find the
cases enjoyable and stimulating.

London 1993

P.S.S.
S.K.
D.J.S.
P.D.W.

Introduction

The MRCP has a reputation of being a difficult examination but, provided it is approached sensibly, one can save an enormous amount of time and effort by concentrating on the subjects that lend themselves to this form of examination. A brief review of former papers shows that some topics appear more often than others and it is vital that any candidate has complete competence in these subjects before extending his knowledge to minutiae which can be largely irrelevant in the success or failure at the examination. Examiners tell us that the examination is designed to test clinical wisdom, insight and practicality rather than an encyclopaedic knowledge. Many people fail themselves by simple ignorance of basic facts or by saying or doing stupid things that indicate a lack of understanding of elementary principles and common sense. The first precept, therefore, is to have a sound basic knowledge and to be able to apply this to clinical problems.

Our book provides a series of cases for revision for Part II of the examination. These hundred cases are all based on actual patients and are of a similar standard and format to those that one expects to meet in the examination. It is the intention that the problems will assess one's knowledge of a subject and indicate deficiencies or areas that need further attention. They are all 'grey' cases and as such are open to different interpretations. In the synopsis of each case those answers that we consider would be most acceptable are printed in bold letters. Obviously some answers are more important than others and would gain more marks. However, these cases are 'grey' and you may arrive at different conclusions but, if so, you must be able to substantiate your reasoning carefully.

Whilst these case histories are directed to the papers, they represent the type of patient that you might expect to face in the clinical section. This is the part of the examination where skill and technique are paramount and in which there is no substitute for practice and experience.

Case 1

A 20-year-old medical student presented with a 12-hour history of fever, vomiting, diarrhoea and severe myalgia. Three weeks previously she had suffered an episode of cystitis which had settled following a five-day course of oral trimethoprim. She took only the oral contraceptive pill and a recent menstrual period was normal. She was a non-smoker, drank little alcohol, and her two flatmates were well. She had not eaten any unusual meals, nor had she travelled abroad.

On examination she looked ill, with a temperature of 39°C. Her pulse rate was 130/min regular, blood pressure 65/40 mmHg, venous pressure not elevated. She had a normal conscious level and no meningism or photophobia. There was a diffuse macular erythema of the trunk and thighs. Marked tenderness of all limb muscles was noted. Abdominal examination revealed no masses or peritonism, and rectal examination showed liquid brown stool, negative for blood. Examination of the nervous, respiratory and cardiovascular systems was otherwise unremarkable.

Investigations: Hb 12.3 g/dl, WBC 28 × 10^9/l, platelets 80 × 10^9/l, thrombin time 22 s (control 15 s), partial thromboplastin time 50 s (control 35 s), fibrin degradation products (FDPs) significantly raised. Urine, stool and blood cultures negative, urea and electrolytes and chest X-ray normal.

1. What is the most likely diagnosis? Suggest two other possibilities.
2. Suggest two further investigations.
3. What further essential feature of the examination would you like to know?
4. What is the treatment?

In a young woman presenting with an abrupt onset of fever, myalgia, rash and shock following a recent menstrual period, with evidence of disseminated intravascular coagulation and sterile blood and urine cultures **toxic shock syndrome** is the likeliest diagnosis. A **septicaemia** is a possibility, for example with a Gram-negative organism following a recent urinary tract infection, although this appeared to have settled following treatment. Meningococcaemia is unlikely but not impossible in the absence of meningism and with negative blood culture. **Food poisoning** is possible, for example due to *Staphylococcus aureus*-produced heat-stable enterotoxin. This may cause abrupt onset of vomiting but fever is usually below 38°C and diarrhoea and rash are uncommon.

Toxic shock syndrome is caused by a staphylococcal exotoxin, 'toxic shock syndrome toxin-1' (TSST-1). This affects predominantly women who use tampons although cases have been reported in men and children. TSST-1 damages vascular endothelium and triggers release of vasoactive agents from platelets and leucocytes. This increases vascular permeability and contributes to tissue damage. As the syndrome is caused by a toxin, blood cultures are often negative although staphylococci may be cultured from a **high vaginal swab**. **Creatine kinase** may be elevated, and a **muscle biopsy** may show a myocytis. **Anti-TSST-1 antibodies** may be detected in low concentration, but this test is not readily available.

A **vaginal examination** is mandatory in this case to look for a tampon and carry out a high vaginal swab.

Treatment is **supportive**. There is as yet no specific anti-TSST-1 antitoxin for therapeutic use. A monoclonal antibody, 'centotoxin' (HA-1A monoclonal antibody to endotoxin), is available for clinical use in conditions due to Gram-negative endotoxin. Trials have demonstrated a reduced mortality in critically ill patients with Gram-negative septicaemia, but centotoxin is of no benefit in toxic shock syndrome. Agents active against Gram-positive toxins are being developed. Antibiotics with anti-staphylococcal activity, such as **vancomycin** or **flucloxacillin** are often given. Mortality remains at approximately 10%.

The risks of toxic shock syndrome are now emphasized by leaflets issued in packets of tampons. The risks are reduced by avoidance of perfumed tampons and by regular changing of tampons.

Case 2

A girl of 16 years with a long history of school refusal began to vomit each Monday morning during her mathematics class and was referred to a child psychiatrist. She subsequently developed an abnormal appetite; on some days she refused to eat, while on others she craved snacks such as potato crisps and instant soups. She lost her interest in physical fitness and stopped jogging each day. She lived with her parents, both schoolteachers, and younger brother, and denied taking drugs or alcohol. She had normal developmental milestones and had been fully immunized as a child. Her menarche occured at the age of 12. She had an appendicectomy at the age of 15.

Two months later, two days before an important examination, she was brought to casualty as she had vomited all food and drink that she had taken for 24 hours. She also had a sore throat and runny nose.

On examination, her temperature was 37.2°C, dry mucus membranes. Pulse rate was 110/min, regular, and blood pressure was 95/60 mmHg lying and 65/40 standing. The rest of the examination was normal.

Investigations: Hb 13 g/dl, WBC 14 × 10^9/l, platelets 269 × 10^9/l, sodium 129 mmol/l, potassium 5.2 mmol/l, urea 8.7 mmol/l, creatinine 56 μmol/l, glucose 2.1 mmol/l. Amylase, chest and abdominal X-rays and ECG normal.

1. What is the diagnosis?
2. Suggest confirmatory investigations.
3. What treatment should be given?
4. Why was she vomiting during her mathematics classes?

This young girl has had episodic vomiting and now presents at a time of stress with a prolonged episode associated with postural hypotension, hyponatraemia, hyperkalaemia, a raised urea but normal creatinine and glucose at the lower limit of normal. These features are all consistent with a diagnosis of **Addison's disease (hypoadrenalism)**. This is uncommon in this age group; typical features such as pigmentation of buccal mucosa and scars may be absent. The symptoms are often vague—weakness, lethargy, anorexia—although an Addisonian crisis may be precipitated by stress, concurrent illness or infection. The most common electrolyte disturbance is a raised urea; sodium and potassium are often normal unless there is a crisis. The vomiting episodes each Monday morning were probably due to relative adrenocortical insufficiency during a stressful class.

The hypoadrenalism may be primary, the most common cause being **autoimmune adrenalitis** or secondary to hypothalamic—pituitary disease or withdrawal of long-term corticosteroid therapy. Other primary causes include **tuberculosis** and rarer causes such as infiltration by tumour or amyloid, or adrenal haemorrhage/infarction as in *Meningococcal septicaemia*.

If the patient is seriously ill, i.v. hydrocortisone should be given, together with saline and glucose, ideally after a blood sample is taken for later **cortisol** and **adrenocorticotrophic hormone** (ACTH) assay. Investigations after the patient has been stabilized include a **short Synacthen test**. Tetracosactrin is given i.m. and plasma cortisol is assayed at time 0, +30 and +60 minutes; an absent or impaired response suggests primary adrenal failure. A high 0900 h ACTH level with low simultaneous cortisol confirms the diagnosis. **Anti-adrenal antibodies** should be assayed. The adrenal glands are best imaged by **magnetic resonance imaging (MRI)**. Secondary hypoadrenalism should be investigated with full **pituitary function tests** and **pituitary computerized axial tomography** or MRI scan.

Long-term treatment is with glucocorticoid and mineralocorticoid, the latter usually as fludrocortisone. Adequacy of treatment with the former is judged by clinical well-being and cortisol levels if hydrocortisone is the replacement agent; fludrocortisone replacement is monitored by absence of postural hypotension and normal plasma renin. Patients should carry a steroid card, wear a Medic-Alert bracelet and keep an emergency supply of hydrocortisone at home.

Case 3

A 57-year-old bus driver of West Indian origin was referred to neurology outpatients with a four-month history of progressive difficulty in walking. He now found it difficult to walk upstairs and was limited by weakness rather than pain. He had no other neurological symptoms. He arrived in Britain from Barbados at the age of 28 and had not returned since. His mother had suffered a similar illness and was now wheelchair bound. He smoked 30 cigarettes a day, took no medications, and drank no alcohol.

Examination revealed a fit-looking man who was right-handed. Neurological examination of the cranial nerves and upper limbs was normal, and neck and back movements were full and painless. Tone was bilaterally increased in both legs and there was weakness in a pyramidal distribution. Reflexes were brisk with ankle and knee clonus and both plantars were extensor. Sensation was normal as was co-ordination, although testing was difficult because of weakness. Romberg's sign negative. General examination was normal.

Investigations: full blood count, urea and electrolytes, glucose, liver and thyroid function, B12 and folate all normal. Syphilis serology negative. ECG showed sinus rhythm with electrical LVH, chest X-ray and X-rays of cervical and lumbar spine normal.

1. Suggest three possible diagnoses.
2. Suggest four useful further investigations.

This case raises the differential diagnosis of progressive spastic paraparesis, suggesting bilateral upper motor neurone lesions affecting the legs. The level of the lesions may be at any point between cerebral cortex and the synapse with lower motor neurones in the cord. The arms and cranial nerves are spared as are bladder and bowel. There are no sensory signs. **Multiple sclerosis** is possible, particularly in a younger patient, although it is extremely unlikely to occur in a person of West Indian origin unless there is some Caucasian (often Celtic) ancestry. The patient arrived in Britain at the age of 28 and would therefore have the low risk of developing MS associated with his place of birth. **Tropical spastic paraparesis** is a much more likely diagnosis in this man. This is due to infection with human T-cell lymphotrophic virus-1 (HTLV-1), a retrovirus which causes a paraparesis, and there is often a family history, as in this case. In Japan, HTLV-1 causes a leukaemia. **Compression of the spinal cord** is possible although some sensory signs would be expected. Subacute combined degeneration of the cord would have associated posterior column signs, and B12 and folate are normal: similarly, **syphilis** causing taboparesis or generalized paralysis of the insane is excluded by negative serology. There are no clinical features to suggest syringomyelia. **Motor neurone disease** is a possibility, as is a **parasagittal meningioma**.

Investigations should include **anti-HTLV-1 antibodies** and **Contrast-enhanced CT brain scan** which may show a meningioma or periventricular plaques. If available, **magnetic resonance imaging (MRI)** is the investigation of choice to exclude compression or an intrinsic lesion causing paraparesis, and may show high signals associated with demyelination. MRI scanning should involve the entire spinal cord and the brain, where it is far superior to CT scanning, especially in defining the posterior fossa and brainstem. **Evoked potentials** (visual, auditory and somatosensory) may also give evidence of demyelination. **Cerebrospinal fluid** examination for **oligoclonal bands** and protein and for anti-HTLV-1 antibodies may be necessary, as may **myelography** in the further pursuit of spinal cord compression.

The diagnosis in this case was **tropical spastic paraparesis**.

Case 4

A 74-year-old widow was referred to the out-patient department for investigation. She had been found to be hypertensive four months previously and had been managed by her general practitioner with a diuretic and a small dose of propranolol. Because of postural hypotension, this treatment had been stopped one month later and her GP had encouraged her to lose weight while carefully observing her blood pressure. Two months before admission she had been found wandering around the house in a confused state by her daughter with whom she lived. By the next morning she was better and her doctor ascribed the attack to transient cerebral ischaemia. At this time, her blood pressure was noted to be 180/105 mmHg and her doctor restarted her on bendrofluazide 5 mg daily. She was well for several weeks, but her daughter noticed her becoming forgetful and losing interest in her grandchildren, on one occasion forgetting their names. There were no other symptoms apart from her longstanding constipation for which she took a proprietary laxative.

On examination, she was moderately obese. Her blood pressure was 175/105 mmHg sitting and standing; pulse rate was 70 per minute and regular. Heart sounds were normal and there was no evidence of cardiac failure. Her fundi showed grade II hypertensive changes. The chest and abdomen were normal. Examination of her central nervous system revealed that she was rather depressed, but answered questions slowly but accurately. Her reflexes were bilaterally brisk, but there was no focal weakness. Vibration sense was diminished at both ankles, but other sensory modalities were normal. Both plantar responses were extensor.

Investigations showed: Hb 12.0 g/dl, WBC 4.8 × 10⁹/l, ESR 29 mm/h, MCV 86 fl. Sodium 133 mmol/l, potassium 3.8 mmol/l, urea 7.8 mmol/l. Random blood glucose 8.7 mmol/l, calcium 2.34 mmol/l. Chest and skull X-rays were normal. Syphilis serology was negative. Her ECG showed some T-wave flattening in V4–V6, but was otherwise normal.

1. What is the diagnosis?
2. How would you confirm this?
3. What treatment would you give?

This lady presents with mild hypertension and mental changes. The mental state appears to fluctuate with disorientation, mild dementia and apparent depression. Her metabolic screen is unremarkable and neurological examination revealed no localizing signs. Impaired vibration sense is a common finding in the elderly, and is usually of no significance. The previous history of hypertension is important as the long term consequences of uncontrolled hypertension include dementia, although it does not normally fluctuate. Drug therapy is a common cause of confusion in the elderly, often due to electrolyte imbalance. This, however, is not the case here and bendrofluazide is a relatively innocuous drug. However, the patient may well have fallen and sustained a head injury following an episode of postural hypotension and not reported it or forgotten about it. The normal haemoglobin and MCV makes the diagnosis of pernicious anaemia extremely unlikely. However, a serum B12 should be requested and likewise, thyroid function tests routinely performed, even though she has very little on examination to suggest thyroid disease.

The most likely diagnosis in this lady is a **subdural haematoma** and should be confirmed by **CT brain scan**. The collection may appear as isodense with brain and may easily be missed, especially if there is no obvious midline shift or ventricular compression. Contrast-enhancement of the scan improves the diagnostic accuracy. A **technetium brain scan** and **bilateral carotid angiography** can be performed, but are now less common as CT scanning is becoming more readily available. **Magnetic resonance imaging** (**MRI scan**) can also be used to diagnose a subdural haematoma. Digital subtraction angiography (DSA) involving a venous injection of contrast is associated with lower morbidity than carotid angiography. An EEG may be normal or may show generalized flattening of electrical activity over one hemisphere. The absence of a skull fracture or history of head injury do not exclude the diagnosis and signs of raised intracranial pressure are often absent until a late stage. 15% of subdural haematomas are bilateral and may account for the non-lateralizing nature of the reflex changes.

There is probably no place for conservative management and bilateral burr holes should be performed and the clot aspirated. If the lesion is large and of long standing, a skull flap should be turned and the lesion removed piecemeal. Subdural haematomas are frequently recurrent in the elderly.

Case 5

A 45-year-old oil executive presented to casualty with a severe epistaxis. He was normally well and when seen had a blood pressure of 115/75 mmHg. The epistaxis was treated by nasal packing.

Eight weeks later he returned to casualty looking sun-tanned, having spent a month working in the Middle East. Whilst there he had developed anorexia, fever, weight loss, with, more recently, a non-productive cough and progressive dyspnoea. In addition, he complained of pain in the left shoulder which was exacerbated by movement.

On examination, he looked unwell and had a temperature of 37.7°C. Pulse was 130 per minute and regular, of normal character. Blood pressure was 100/60 mmHg, JVP + 4 cm. The cardiac apex was slightly displaced laterally, but was not hyperdynamic. On auscultation, the first heart sound could not be heard, but there was a prominent third heart sound. At the left sternal edge a short medium pitched early diastolic murmur was heard with a soft ejection systolic murmur. At the apex there was a soft mid-diastolic murmur. He was dyspnoeic at rest and had bilateral basal crepitations in his chest. There was no lymphadenopathy but his spleen could just be tipped.

Initial investigations showed: Hb 10.6 g/dl, WBC 10.7 × 10/l, ESR 76 mm/h. Platelets 256 × 10⁹/l, clotting studies normal. Chest X-ray showed a normal sized heart and pronounced pulmonary congestion. X-rays of his left shoulder were normal. ECG showed sinus rhythm with episodes of Wenckebach heart block. There was T-wave inversion in the left precordial leads. Urinalysis showed 1 + of blood.

1. What is the diagnosis?
2. Suggest two important investigations.
3. What is the cause of his rhythm change?
4. What is the probable cause of his shoulder pain?
5. What would be your management?

This young man has the physical signs of **acute severe aortic regurgitation** and his fever, anaemia, raised ESR, splenomegaly, and microscopic haematuria suggest **infective endocarditis** as the cause. His nasal packing was perhaps the source of infection.

The signs of acute severe aortic regurgitation differ from those of chronic disease. The regurgitant blood enters a non-dilated ventricle and end-diastolic pressure rises dramatically, causing early mitral valve closure and is recognized clinically by the absent first heart sound and the short length of the early diastolic murmur. The velocity of left ventricular contraction is not increased and hence the cardiac apex is not hyperdynamic and the pulse is of normal character. The high LVEDP means the diastolic blood pressure is not significantly lowered and the pulse pressure is not widened. His apical mid-diastolic murmur is an Austin Flint murmur. **Blood Cultures** (at least 6 sets) and **echocardiography** should be carried out. The latter may be **transthoracic** or **transoesophageal**.

Rhythm disturbances are by no means rare in endocarditis of the aortic valve and are due to **extravalvular extension of infection** into the conducting tissue. Complete heart block may be produced and a pacemaker may be necessary.

A retrospective study of bacterial endocarditis showed almost half to have musculo-skeletal symptoms, usually arthralgia, myalgia or low back pain. In 27% these were amongst the first symptoms of the disease. The symptoms are perhaps due to **circulating immune complexes**. An infective arthritis is another, less likely, possibility with this man.

Management of this patient must include **high dose intravenous antibiotics** started immediately after several blood cultures have been taken. Until an organism is grown, and sensitivities known, treatment is usually commenced with an aminoglycoside, such as gentamicin and a penicillin. He will require early **aortic valve replacement**. The hazards of placing a valve into an infected position must be weighed against the risks of his continuing severe valvular incompetence and optimal timing of surgery requires experience and judgement. Postoperatively a full course of antibiotic therapy must be completed.

Case 6

A 46-year-old petrol pump attendant was admitted as an emergency. He had smoked 20 cigarettes a day for many years, but apart from several episodes of acute bronchitis had always been well. Ten days previously he had become ill with generalized weakness, anorexia and a dry cough. His own doctor had prescribed tetracycline and he had started to feel a little better despite a worsening cough and increasing exertional dyspnoea. Two days before admission, he had developed diarrhoea and on the day of admission he became confused.

On admission to hospital he was cyanosed, febrile (38.5°C) and disorientated. Blood pressure was 125/78 mmHg, pulse 110 beats per minute, regular, with no evidence of heart failure. The breath sounds were diminished at both bases with widespread inspiratory crackles to the midzone and bronchial breathing at the right base. There were no abnormalities of the abdomen or focal neurological signs.

Investigations: Hb 12.9 g/dl, WBC 9.0 × 10^9/l (93% polymorphs, 6% lymphocytes, 1% eosinophils). Platelets 120 × 10^9/l, ESR 86 mm/hr. Sodium 129 mmol/l, potassium, 4.3 mmol/l, urea 5.9 mmol/l, random blood glucose 6.8 mmol/l. Liver function tests: albumin 28 g/l, aspartate transaminase 60 U/l; bilirubin 12 μmol/l HBD 190 U/l, alkaline phosphatase 145 U/l. Chest X-ray showed widespread shadowing in both lung fields with relative sparing of the apices and consolidation at the right base. Blood gases—PO_2 7.9 kPa (59 mmHg), PCO_2 4.7 kPa (35 mmHg), pH 7.39. Electrocardiogram showed a sinus tachycardia.

He was thought to have widespread bronchopneumonia and was started on intravenous ampicillin and flucloxacillin. The next day his condition markedly deteriorated with increasing dyspnoea, confusion and cyanosis. ECG showed no change and blood gases showed a PO_2 of 6.4 kPa (48 mmHg), PCO_2 4.8 kPa (36 mmHg), and pH 7.36. Repeat chest X-ray showed increased shadowing in both lung fields and early involvement of the right apex.

1. What is the diagnosis?
2. How would you confirm this and give four other useful investigations?

The patient has an acute severe pneumonia with a prodromal illness that has failed to respond to several antibiotics. This raises the possibility of an atypical infective agent. His sudden deterioration could have been caused by a worsening of his pneumonia, a pneumothorax, massive pulmonary collapse or even a pulmonary embolus. A repeat chest X-ray and blood gases would help to distinguish these. Further attempts to isolate the organism would be made and include **blood cultures** and **bronchoscopy** or **transtracheal aspiration of sputum** in the event of a non-productive cough. **Serum for viral antibodies** could include the commoner viruses or 'atypical' agents including *Mycoplasma pneumoniae* and psittacosis.

This man has not responded to tetracycline which makes a diagnosis of Mycoplasma and psittacosis unlikely. He does have a relatively low white cell count with lymphopenia, mildly abnormal LFTs, diarrhoea and a degree of confusion out of proportion to his hypoxia or hyponatraemia. These features are all typical of **legionnaires' disease**, and the diagnosis is confirmed by the development of **antibodies to** *Legionella pneumophilia* during the course of the illness. Because seroconversion takes up to two weeks, the diagnosis must be made clinically if effective treatment is to be started early. It is now possible to culture the organism on special media, although this is difficult. Other features of the disease include a relative bradycardia, pleurisy, hypophosphataemia, abnormal liver function tests, gastrointestinal symptoms, confusion, proteinuria and a mild coagulopathy. This patient has low platelets and a **clotting screen** including fibrin degradation products should be performed.

Treatment is usually with erythromycin and/or rifampicin. Clinical improvement may take up to a week following the commencement of therapy. A smaller percentage of patients respond to tetracycline but this can no longer be regarded as the treatment of choice.

Case 7

A 47-year-old housewife was referred to the dermatology clinic with a complaint of generalized pruritis for one year. This had started insidiously but had recently become troublesome, keeping her awake at night. She otherwise felt well, with a good appetite and steady weight, but did admit to a dry mouth. She did not smoke, drank occasionally and was on no medication. No other members of her family had experienced itching.

On examination, she looked well and was not anaemic, jaundiced, cyanosed or clubbed. There was no lymphadenopathy. There were scattered scratch marks, but no other skin lesions were seen. Cardiovascular and respiratory systems normal. In her abdomen, the liver was palpable two finger breadths below the costal margin. No other masses were palpable and the spleen could not be felt. Urinalysis was negative.

Investigations: Hb 13.7 g/dl (normal film), WBC 5.8 × 10⁹/l, sodium 137 mmol/l, potassium 4.2 mmol/l, bicarbonate 24 mmol/l, urea 5.2 mmol/l, aspartate transaminase 36 U/l, bilirubin 12 μ mol/l, protein 64 g/l, albumin 37 g/l, alkaline phosphatase 470 U/l, calcium 2.35 mmol/l, phosphate 0.80 mmol/l, fasting glucose 4.5 mmol/l, thyroxine 125 mmol/l. Chest X-ray normal.

1. What is the most likely diagnosis?
2. How would you confirm this?
3. What treatment would you give?

This lady raises the differential diagnosis of pruritis. There is no evidence of specific skin disease and so a systemic cause is suggested. Malignancy can present in this way, but her history is long and there is no evidence on examination. Similarly a reticulosis or myeloproliferative disorder is unlikely. Her investigations exclude uraemia, diabetes, myxoedema, hyperthyroidism or jaundice as causes.

Her one abnormal investigation is the raised alkaline phosphatase and this suggests the diagnosis of **primary biliary cirrhosis**. Approximately 50% of patients with this disease present with pruritis and most sufferers develop this symptom at some stage during their disease. The pruritis may be present for some years before jaundice develops.

Although the diagnosis is also suggested by finding a high level of serum IgM or a positive anti-mitochondrial antibody titre, which is present in over 95% of sufferers, confirmation is obtained by **liver biopsy**. In the early stages bile duct damage is shown by swelling and proliferation of epithelial cells and the ducts are surrounded by a dense inflammatory infiltrate of lymphocytes and plasma cells with epitheloid cells and a few eosinophils. Granulomata may be seen. Later the lesions become more widespread, although less specific, and fibrosis occurs ending in cirrhosis.

Pruritis can be treated with cholestyramine, although this is unpalatable, and antihistamines and phenobarbitone may help as may norethandrolone, although this deepens jaundice. Supplements of fat-soluble vitamins, calcium and phosphate should be given in view of malabsorption. In view of the possible immunological aetiology, immunosuppressive therapy has been tried; azathioprine and corticosteroids have been tried but without benefit, the latter containdicated because of osteoporosis. Penicillamine should not be given in the early stages, but may improve survival in advanced cases due to its immunological, chelating and antifibrotic effects. Colchicine has been shown to improve outcome and some suggest phototherapy; early results with cyclosporin A are promising.

The prognosis is variable; those with no symptoms or pruritis alone may survive for twenty years, while those with jaundice may die within five years of liver failure or bleeding varices. **Liver transplantation** is now frquently carried out, in particular in patients with bilirubin in excess of 100 μ mol/l, and this has improved the prognosis.

Case 8

A 28-year-old woman, 16 weeks into her first pregnancy, was brought into casualty by her husband following a collapse in her bathroom. She had been troubled since the fifth week of her pregnancy by daily, severe vomiting. One week prior to this presentation, she had been admitted by the obstetricians and treated with intravenous antiemetics and a dextrose–saline infusion with potassium supplements. Following this, her vomiting had improved but she had become increasingly confused and unsteady on her feet, and on the day of admission had collapsed while climbing out of the bath. She had not lost consciousness or fitted, and her husband did not think she had injured her head. She was taking Pregaday, a combined iron and folate preparation, and unfortunately had continued to smoke 10 cigarettes daily.

On examination she was conscious and co-operative but was disorientated in time and place and was frightened. She had poor short-term recall. She had no meningism or photophobia. She was afebrile. Blood pressure 120/160 mmHg. Abnormalities were confined to the nervous system. There was a suggestion of lateral nystagmus on horizontal gaze, and her pupils were small, equal and reacted very sluggishly to light. Fundoscopy revealed small bilateral retinal haemorrhages but no papilloedema. The cranial nerves were otherwise normal. Limbs displayed normal tone and power but her reflexes were less brisk than expected and she had a strong bilateral plantar withdrawal response. Poor finger–nose co-ordination was evident. She was very unsteady on standing, swaying in all directions. Romberg's test was negative.

Investigations: full blood count, film, clotting screen, liver function tests and calcium normal. Urea 2.4 mmol/l, sodium 134 mmol/l, potassium 3.3 mmol/l, creatinine 60 μmol/l, random glucose 4.9 mmol/l, bicarbonate 28 mmol/l. ECG and chest X-ray normal. Contrast-enhanced CT brain scan normal. CSF examination revealed: opening pressure 17 cmCSF clear and colourless, red cells 5/mm³, no white cells, protein 0.28 g/l, glucose 3.1 mmol/l.

1. What is the diagnosis?
2. Suggest a useful further investigation.
3. What is the treatment?
4. Why has her condition deteriorated?

This young woman gives a long history of vomiting, and now has a triad of a confusional state, cerebellar ataxia and ocular abnormalities comprising nystagmus, abnormal pupillary reaction to light and retinal haemorrhages. The diagnosis is **Wernicke's encephalopathy** due to dietary deficiency of thiamine, vitamin B1. Other diagnoses to be considered are **raised intracranial pressure** for example due to a space-occupying lesion such as a **tumour** (meningiomas in particular often enlarge during pregnancy) or **benign intracranial hypertension**. The CT brain scan and CSF findings are against these. An **encephalitis**, for example due to herpes simplex is possible, although the CSF again is not supportive and CT often shows low-density lesions in the temporal lobes. Multiple sclerosis rarely presents this dramatically with impaired consciousness; a drug reaction to antiemetics is also unlikely to last this long.

Wernicke's encephalopathy more often affects alcoholics who have poor diets; other vitamin deficiency syndromes may co-exist (e.g. scurvy). Other features of thiamine deficiency include ocular palsy, peripheral neuropathy and Korsakoff's psychosis which may result in coma and even treated still results in a high mortality. Thiamine deficiency may also cause beri-beri with heart failure. The diagnosis is made clinically and confirmed by reduced in vitro **red blood cell transketolase** activity, which may increase by the addition of thiamine. Clinical response to **thiamine**, given orally or parenterally is often dramatic and may be useful diagnostically.

The cause of this patient's deterioration is likely to be the treatment she was given with intravenous glucose. Many enzyme systems involved in glucose metabolism, such as in the glycolytic pathway are thiamine-dependant. In thiamine deficiency, administration of glucose results in shunting to other pathways with the generation of neurotoxic metabolites.

Prolonged vomiting during pregnancy may be fatal, as in untreated hyperemesis gravidarum. It may also indicate the presence of a hydatidiform mole.

Case 9

A 25-year-old woman presented to medical out-patients with a three-month history of increasing thirst and polyuria. During this time she had put on two stone in weight. Four months previously she had had a mastoid operation and subsequently developed irregular periods.

There was no other past medical history of note and in her family history one sister had been treated for thyrotoxicosis.
Examination was entirely normal.

Investigations showed: urea and electrolytes, calcium and phosphate, glucose tolerance test—all normal. Mid-stream urine showed no growth.

1. Give two possible diagnoses.
2. Describe the test which would distinguish between these. Are any hazards associated with this test?
3. Give three further investigations.

This young woman either has **diabetes insipidus** or **compulsive water drinking**. Her normal glucose tolerance test excludes diabetes mellitus and her normal calcium and potassium rule out the common causes of renal tubular damage which may give rise to polyuria.

A formal fluid deprivation test measuring urine and serum osmolalities, with regular weighing in hospital under observation, will show if she can concentrate her urine. The test can be hazardous due to excessive loss of fluid and should be terminated if the subject loses more than 3% of initial body weight or more than 3 l urine is passed. An injection of synthetic antidiuretic hormone (DDAVP) should be given at the end of the test to see if exogenous ADH causes urine concentration, as would be expected in pituitary causes of diabetes insipidus where there is lack of antidiuretic hormone.

This woman failed to concentrate her urine during fluid deprivation, but did so after injection of DDAVP, proving pituitary diabetes insipidus. Though in the majority of patients no underlying cause can be found, it is important to exclude a pituitary tumour. She should have a pituitary X-ray, **computerized axial tomography** (**CT**) of the pituitary fossa, and **magnetic resonance imaging** (**MRI scan**) as well as having her visual fields assessed.

Head trauma may precede the development of diabetes insipidus, though there is no history of this here. Rarer causes include granulomatous disease and local infections, including basal meningitis. Any relationship of her developing diabetes insipidus with her previous mastoid surgery remains only speculative.

Treatment is with DDAVP which can be given intranasally or intravenously.

Case 10

A 17-year-old girl was referred for investigation of amenorrhoea. Her mother said that breast development had started at the age of 10, but she had never had a menstrual period, while her mother's menarche was at age 12. She had more body hair than was usual in her family. She had occasional frontal headaches, took no medications and drank no alcohol. She was vegetarian. Her family had emigrated from Pakistan when she was nine. She was the eldest of four children, and the only girl. She had a periumbilical hernia repaired at the age of 18 months. She was progressing well at school, studying for four 'A' levels and hoping to go to university to study law. In private, she revealed that she had a boyfriend and normal sexual drive, but had never engaged in sexual intercourse.

Examination revealed a well-looking girl. She was of normal height and weight for her age and sex. There was hirsutism and a small symmetrical goitre. The external genitalia were normal with no clitoromegaly. The hymen was not imperforate. Breast development was complete. The rest of the examination was normal.

Investigations: urea and electrolytes, full blood count, glucose and liver function tests normal. Urinary pregnancy test negative. Skull X-ray showed normal pituitary fossa. The levels of the following hormones are shown (with normal ranges in brackets):

Oestradiol:	115 pmol/l	(follicular 15–120, luteal 100–340)
Testosterone:	31 nmol/l	(< 5)
LH:	32 IU/l	(follicular 4–30, mid-cycle 50–150, luteal 3–4)
FSH:	4 IU/l	(follicular 4–30, mid-cycle 15–50, luteal 4–15)
Prolactin:	280 mU/l	(20–360)
TSH:	2.5 mU/l	(0.8–5.0)
Thyroxine:	125 nmol/l	(60–140)

1. What is the likeliest diagnosis? Suggest two alternatives.
2. Suggest four useful investigations.
3. How would you treat this girl?

This girl presents with primary amenorrhoea. Pregnancy and an imperforate hymen have been excluded, as has ovarian failure both by normal development of breasts and external genitalia and by a normal serum oestradiol. The combination of hirsutism with amenorrhoea suggests androgen excess, confirmed by an elevated testosterone level. She does not have features of virilization such as clitoromegaly, acne or frontal balding. The levels of LH and prolactin are normal with low–normal FSH, and a high LH: FSH ratio. This suggests the likeliest diagnosis of **polycystic ovary syndrome** (**PCOS**). Obesity is not invariable. In a more severe form, hirsutes and virilization may occur due to excessive androgen secretion from multiple ovarian cysts and the adrenal glands (Stein–Leventhal Syndrome). Another important diagnosis to consider is **congenital adrenal hyperplasia** (**CAH**), caused by a defect in the steroid biosynthetic pathway, most commonly 21-hydroxylase. This reduces cortisol production with a resultant rise in ACTH and diversion of precursors into the production of testosterone. Severe cases often present at birth with adrenal failure and sexual ambiguity but mild cases may go undetected and present with primary amenorrhoea and hirsutes. An **androgen-secreting tumour**, adrenal or ovarian, is possible though less likely since levels of testosterone are often much higher and virilization occurs. Finally, she does not have the clinical features of Cushing's syndrome which can present this way.

Investigations include **ovarian ultrasound** which showed ovaries with thickened capsules, multiple ovarian cysts up to 5 mm diameter and an echobright stroma, typical of PCOS. Uterine presence was confirmed since absence is a rare cause of primary amenorrhoea. **Gonadothrophin releasing hormone** may by given i.v., and typically an exaggerated release of LH occurs. **Sex-hormone binding globulin** (**SHBG**) levels are low. **Ovarian biopsy** can be carried out at **laparoscopy**. In CAH, levels of ACTH, **17-hydroxyprogesterone** and **urinary pregnanetriol** are raised. Treatment of PCOS is aimed at hirsutism, regularisation of periods and fertility. **Oestrogens** or the **oral contaceptive pill** raise SHBG levels and lower free androgens. **Prednisolone** given in a reversed circadian manner may help hirsutes. **Clomiphene or tamoxifen** given days 2–6 of the cycle then HCG on day 12 can help fertility. **Resection of cysts** may be necessary.

Case 11

A 41-year-old Indian woman presented with a five-year history of persistent low back pain previously treated unsuccessfully by an orthopaedic department. Eighteen months previously she had had a partial thyroidectomy for a non-toxic goitre.

Examination failed to reveal any physical abnormalities.

Investigations showed Hb 10.0 g/dl, serum calcium 1.9 mmol/l, phosphate 0.74 mmol/l, alkaline phosphatase 200 U/l. Blood urea and electrolytes normal. Serum albumin 35 g/l.

1. Suggest three possible causes for her biochemical abnormality.
2. What five additional investigations are indicated?
3. What treatment would you recommend for her back pain?

The combination of hypocalcaemia and hypophosphataemia in this case points to a diagnosis of **osteomalacia** due to **dietary deficiency of calcium, lack of vitamin D** or **intestinal disease with malabsorption**, such as tropical sprue, and in these conditions the alkaline phosphatase is usually elevated. Osteomalacia, which may be caused by any of these diagnoses, is particularly common in immigrants from India and Pakistan. Here there may be a multifactorial cause of dietary vitamin D deficiency, including pigmentation of skin resulting in the synthesis of less endogenous vitamin D and calcium binding by phytate from chappatis in their diet.

Post-thyroidectomy hypoparathyroidism is rare and is usually associated with hypocalcaemia in combination with hyperphosphataemia.

Investigations must include **bone X-rays** which may show demineralization and Looser's zones. Plasma 25-hydroxyvitamin D can be assayed. **Bone biopsy** which will show excess osteoid, is uncomfortable and rarely carried out. **Urinary excretion** of **calcium** should be determined; although low in most cases of hypocalcaemia, it is elevated in two uncommon conditions, namely renal tubular acidosis and essential hypercalciuria. Small bowel malabsorption may be assessed by faecal fat excretion and if indicated, **small bowel biopsy** performed. A **detailed dietary history** is mandatory.

Treatment should be begun with **oral calcium** and 1-α-hydroxy-vitamin D3 (this is a more potent form of vitamin D with a shorter half-life, allowing reasonably rapid changes in dosage). **Back support** may be required temporarily to relieve the pain and dietary advice should, of course, be given.

Case 12

A 77-year-old widower was admitted with two weeks of progressive breathlessness. He was known to the cardiology team who had been looking after him since a Starr–Edwards aortic valve replacement five years previously; his course had been complicated at the time by complete heart block and he had a permanent ventricular pacemaker in place. Eight months before this admission he had suffered an anterior myocardial infarction complicated by post-infarction heart failure. Despite this he was subsequently able to cope well at home and usually managed to walk 200 yards on the flat, limited by breathlessness; when he presented, he was very breathless at rest. He also had a non-productive cough, anorexia and a low-grade fever but no chest pain. Medications on admission: frusemide 80 mg o.d., enalapril 10 mg o.d., amiodarone 200 mg o.d., warfarin 6 mg o.d., allopurinol 100 mg o.d. He still smoked five cigarettes daily and drank no alcohol.

On examination he looked unwell, was thin and centrally cyanosed. He was febrile 37.6°C, pulse 110 regular, BP 120/70 mmHg, venous pressure 5 cm above the sternal angle, no peripheral oedema. The heart sounds were of a competent Starr–Edwards aortic prosthesis. There were bilateral fine inspiratory crackles in both lung fields extending to the upper zones from the bases.

Investigations: EGG unchanged with sinus rhythm with an old Q-wave anterior infarction. Chest X-ray: cardiothoracic ratio 0.7, permanent pacemaker in situ, bilateral fine nodular interstitial shadows especially in the bases and perihilar regions. Full blood count normal, prothrombin ratio 2.8. Urea 10 mmol/l, creatinine 125 μmol/l, electrolytes and liver function tests normal. Blood cultures sterile x 3 sets, serology for *Legionella* and *Mycoplasma* negative. Arterial blood gases on air: PO_2 5.5 kPa (41 mmHg), PCO_2 3.3 kPa (25 mmHg), pH 7.43. Echocardiogram: dilated left ventricle with globally poor systolic function, no valvular abnormality or vegetations. Pacemaker function test satisfactory.

A diagnosis of pulmonary oedema complicated by bronchopneumonia was made. He was given oxygen, physiotherapy, i.v. frusemide, ampicillin and gentamicin and oral metolazone and erythromycin. Despite a 6 l diuresis in the first 48 hours he deteriorated and died five days after admission.

1. Suggest a differential diagnosis. What is the most likely final diagnosis?
2. What would have been the diagnostic investigation and appropriate treatment?

This man with known heart disease presented with severe dyspnoea, non-productive cough and low grade fever. He was severely hypoxic and chest X-ray showed bilateral interstitial shadowing and cardiomegaly. He did not respond to diuretics despite a good diuresis, nor did he respond to broad spectrum antibiotics. Cultures were negative as was serology for *Legionella* and *Mycoplasma*. Lack of response suggests the wrong therapy or the wrong diagnosis. One should not assume a cardiac cause simply because of the previous history of cardiac problems; there was little clinical evidence for heart failure, and non-cardiac causes of his presentation should be considered.

An **atypical pneumonia** is possible with negative early serology but he should have made some response to erythromycin; however, some cases of *Legionella* respond only to rifampicin. A **viral pneumonia** is a possibility; viral titres should have been checked. **Multiple pulmonary emboli** are unlikely since he was adequately anticoagulated. **Lymphangitis carcinomatosa** or **pulmonary haemorrhage** may present in this way as rarely may **non-cardiogenic pulmonary oedema (shock lung syndrome)** although there were no obvious causes of this.

An **alveolitis** with or without **pulmonary fibrosis** can present in precisely this way and is highest on the list of differentials. This may be **cryptogenic** as in Hamann—Rich syndrome, an aggressive and rapidly fatal form of cryptogenic fibrosing alveolitis, or may be an **extrinsic alveolitis**. A drug-induced pneumonitis is possible, and **amiodarone** was felt to be the causative agent in this case, based upon postmortem lung histology. Amiodarone can cause an alveolitis and pneumonitis progressing to fibrosis. Some series suggest that this occurs in 10% of those taking the drug, although most accept a lower rate of 1–5%. It is more likely with higher doses. This side-effect can occur immediately on starting the drug or many months or years later.

The treatment is to **stop amiodarone** and give **corticosteroids**; most cases regress. Early recognition is aided by serial chest X-rays at six or 12-monthly intervals and serial transfer factor estimations. The diagnosis may have been made by **bronchoscopy** and **transbronchial lung biopsy**, although this would have been associated with considerable risk in a patient who was so severely hypoxic.

Case 13

On a cold December day a 64-year-old street trader was brought into casualty by ambulance. His friends said he had fainted suddenly at his stall and had been unconscious for about two minutes. He had turned pale but had not fitted, gone blue or been incontinent. When he came round he was somewhat dazed but well orientated. The patient denied any warning of the faint and said that he now felt quite all right and did not want to come into hospital. He denied any previous attacks but his wife said later that he had fainted four months before while driving his Jaguar car and had done a considerable amount of damage to the car. She had been worried about him but he refused to see a doctor. He was taking no medication and smoked about 25 cigarettes a day; he liked to drink stout with his friends at the market. Fifteen years before he had had bilateral varicose vein ligations.

On examination he was conscious and well orientated. Neurological examination was entirely normal. There were no carotid bruits. Blood pressure was 170/110 mmHg. He had a normal pulse of 80 per minute. There was a systolic ejection murmur along the left sternal edge and scattered crepitations and rhonchi in the lung fields. There were no other physical signs.

Immediate investigations showed Hb 14.9 g/dl, WBC 6.0 × 10⁹/l, ESR 28 mm/h. Chest X-ray—minimal cardiomegaly. ECG—non-specific T-wave flattening in left ventricular leads.

1. What are the two most likely diagnoses?
2. Suggest one other possible diagnosis.
3. What would be the four most useful investigations?

This man has had two transient attacks of loss of consciousness. The history is inadequate to make an accurate diagnosis and great care must be taken to go into the details of each attack.

It is of vital importance to exclude **Stokes–Adam attacks** which can occur despite his normal ECG. This may have occurred acutely following a silent myocardial infarction and his ECG should be repeated together with **cardiac enzymes**. He will also need prolonged monitoring of his ECG by means of a **24 hour tape** to look for rhythm disturbances.

Epilepsy can cause transient loss of consciousness at any age. He is clearly an unreliable historian and so one cannot put too much weight on the absence of an aura. The absence of tonic and clonic phases and the lack of incontinence do not exclude the possibility of a fit. In this man's case a seizure could be alcohol related, due to cerebrovascular disease or related to a secondary bronchial carcinoma. He must have an EEG and a **contrast-enhanced CT brain scan**.

Brain stem ischaemia is less likely without associated symptoms such as vertigo, paraesthesiae or diplopia. It could be due to direct vertebral artery disease or to bony compression. Although degenerative arterial change is the most likely cause, **syphilis serology** should be determined.

Postural hypotension might account for his present attack, especially as it occurred on a cold day when he may well have consumed alcohol. It would not, however, explain the first episode.

Drop attacks, where the patient falls to the ground without warning, are not associated with loss of consciousness and occur almost exclusively in females. They are, therefore, unlikely here.

Hypoglycaemia *must* be excluded in any unconscious patient, but is unlikely to cause such transient attacks.

The aortic ejection murmur, in association with a normal pulse, has no relevance to his attacks. Despite lack of clinical evidence of significant left ventricular outflow obstruction an **echocardiogram** is indicated.

Case 14

A 26-year-old travel agent was brought to casualty by her husband with a cold, painful left hand. This had developed suddenly that day while she was at home. Her health was generally good, although she had suffered a left calf deep venous thrombosis the previous year and had taken warfarin for three months. She and her husband were being investigated for fertility problems following their inability to have a child during their six-year marriage; on three occasions, the patient had suffered miscarriages early in the course of a pregnancy. She was taking no medications, did not smoke or drink alcohol.

Examination revealed a healthy-looking woman in obvious pain. Her left hand was cold and white and neither the radial nor the ulnar pulse could be felt. All other pulses were present, and there were no bruits. The rest of the examination was normal.

Investigations: Hb 12.3 g/dl, WBC 8.6 × 10^9/1, platelets 107 × 10^9/1. Urea and electrolytes, glucose, ECG and chest X-ray normal. Doppler ultrasound examination could detect neither radial nor ulnar pulses on the left side.

1. What is the diagnosis?
2. Suggest four further investigations.
3. Describe three further features associated with this condition.

This young woman has a history of recurrent early foetal loss, deep venous thrombosis and now presents with an acute arterial occlusion affecting the left arm. She is thrombocytopenic. This is suggestive of the **antiphospholipid syndrome**. In 50% of cases this is a primary syndrome, but in 50% there is an association with systemic lupus erythematosus or 'lupus-like disease'. There are detectable **antiphosholipid antibodies** and/or **'lupus anticoagulant'**. The latter is detected by prolongation of three in vitro phospholipid-dependent clotting tests which do not correct with normal plasma: Russell's viper venom test; kaolin–cephalin clotting time; thromboplastin inhibition time. Some patients also have **anti-cardiolipin antibodies** either IgM or IgG, which are also found in association with some malignancies, infections and drugs.

Serological markers for SLE such as **anti-nuclear factor** (**ANF**) and **anti-double stranded DNA antibodies** should be carried out as should **complement activity**.

The extent of this young woman's arterial thrombosis should be investigated by **arteriography** and urgent surgical intervention is necessary to prevent loss of her hand.

The mechanism involved in recurrent foetal loss in this syndrome is uncertain, and it is not clear if these antibodies are pathogenic or if they are disease markers. The associations of the antiphospholipid syndrome are of:

1. Thrombosis, arterial and venous.
2. Recurrent foetal loss, especially before three months gestation.
3. Haematological: thrombocytopenia, Coombs' positive haemolytic anaemia.
4. Dermatological: livedo reticularis, skin nodules/necrosis.
5. Neurological: chorea, transverse myelitis, dementia.

Studies looking at five-year follow-up of patients with antiphospholipid syndrome have shown that there is no correlation between antibody levels and SLE activity, and that immunosuppressant drugs and corticosteroids do not reduce the incidence of further vascular occlusions. Life-long **anticoagulation** with warfarin is necessary and should be substituted for heparin subcutaneously during subsequent pregnancies.

Case 15

A 23-year-old actress was found semiconscious by her flatmate with two empty tablet bottles on her bedside table. That morning she was known to have bought fifty aspirins and had also obtained sixty co-proxamol tablets from her doctor for a strained back. She had been seen by a friend three hours before leaving a coffee bar. On admission she was semicomatose, there was no evidence of external injury and she was hyperventilating and sweating. Her pulse was 110 per minute, blood pressure 100/60 mmHg, chest clear. There were no abnormal signs in the abdomen or in the central nervous system and skull X-ray showed no fractures.

1. What would be the six most important points in the immediate management of this girl?
2. Suggest six complications that may arise from her condition.

The dangers in this case are those specific to salicylate, paracetamol and opiate poisoning, together with the potential hazards in the management of a comatose patient. Emergency treatment is aimed at maintaining the vital functions of adequate ventilation and circulation. Having ensured patency of the airways and assessed that ventilation is inadequate on objective grounds, **intermittent positive pressure ventilation** may be necessary. 100% oxygen should be given if the patient is comatose. **Naloxone** reverses the central depressant effects of opiates and is given if there is respiratory depression; however, the duration of action of naloxone is shorter that the opiates and an infusion may be necessary.

Circulatory failure is treated with intravenous fluids and if necessary inotropic support. Pulse, blood pressure and central venous pressure should be monitored, the latter by a central line. Investigations should include **acid-base status, renal function** and **drug levels** by a **blood** and **urine screen**. In view of the potential hepatotoxicity of paracetamol, **liver function tests** (particularly **clotting**) shold be monitored. A **forced alkaline diuresis** should be initiated if plasma salicylate levels exceed 500 mg/l (3.6 mmol/l) since under alkaline conditions the excretion of salicylates is increased manifold. At salicylate levels lower than 500 mg/l, saline diuresis is adequate.

The hazards of paracetamol poisoning are related to a hepato-toxic metabolite. Sulphydryl donors such as methionine and N-acetylcysteine prevent susequent liver damage by binding to this metabolite. N-acetylcysteine should be given as an infusion if the serum paracetamol level at a given time post-ingestion is above a line connecting 200 mg/l (1.32 mmol/l) at four hours and 10 mg/l at 24 hours. Other therapeutic procedures such as charcoal haemoperfusion are limited to some centres and their efficacy is limited.

Complications of poisoning with these drugs therefore include acid-base and electrolyte disturbances, renal failure, respiratory depression, liver failure, bleeding tendency, gastric erosions, and convulsions.

Hepatocellular failure due to paracetamol occurs three to four days after the overdose. Poor prognostic features include a prothrombin time > 30 seconds at 48 hours or > 50 seconds at 72 hours, and severe acidosis. In these circumstances, **liver transplantation** should be considered.

Case 16

A 28-year-old printer was admitted to hospital severely ill. Eight days previously he had developed a painful swelling in his left axilla for which he had been prescribed ampicillin. This had continued to increase in size over the next six days, after which he became progressively more unwell with fever, anorexia and vomiting on two occasions. On questioning, he thought he had passed less urine than normal and that it had appeared concentrated. Two days before admission he had developed dyspnoea on climbing stairs. There was no significant past medical history, although he had been feeling more easily fatigued in the previous two months.

On examination he was lethargic and pale. His temperature was 38.4°C with warm peripheries. Respiratory rate, 20 per minute; blood pressure 130/90 mmHg; JVP was raised 5 cm and his pulse was 110 beats per minute and regular. The apex beat was palpable in the anterior axillary line and there was a gallop rhythm. Examination of the fundi revealed A-V nipping and vessel tortuosity. There was slight ankle oedema. In the respiratory system, extensive bilateral crepitations were heard. The other systems were normal, apart from the presence of a 6 cm × 8 cm tender, fluctuant abscess in the left axilla.

Investigations showed: Hb 8.0 g/dl, MCV 80 fl; MCHC 19 mmol/l, WBC 18 × 10⁹/l (92% polymorphs), platelets 220 × 10⁹/l, reticulocytes 2%. Sodium 124 mmol/l, potassium 5.8 mmol/l, blood urea 56.6 mmol/l. MSU—10⁶ RBCs/mm³. Protein + +. Urobilinogen—trace. Chest X-ray showed cardiomegaly and pulmonary oedema.

1. What is the diagnosis?
2. What are the two most important steps in management?

This man has acute renal failure as evidenced by a history of oliguria and a raised blood urea occurring during an acute illness. However, he also has a normochromic, normocytic anaemia and evidence of chronic hypertension. This is very suggestive of previous significant renal impairment and that the diagnosis is **acute on chronic renal failure**. Anaemia may occur with acute renal failure, but usually after several weeks and tends to be less severe. Severe haemolysis may in itself cause acute renal failure, but the absence of significant amounts of urobilinogen or a reticulocytosis excludes this.

His immediate problems are **fluid overload** and infection; the former, should large doses of **intravenous diuretics** and **fluid restriction** fail, will require **dialysis**. The choice between peritoneal and haemodialysis is not clear cut, but peritoneal dialysis is effective for patients in whom fluid overload is the predominant problem and when the blood urea is not rising very rapidly. However it is uncomfortable, and peritonitis, chest infections, hypoalbuminaemia and hypovolaemic collapse can easily occur.

His other urgent problem is **sepsis** from his axillary abscess which in this case has probably led to septicaemia and subsequent acute tubular necrosis. This is a common presentation of chronic renal disease where the patient has undiagnosed chronic impairment, develops an intercurrent illness and is followed by a rapid deterioration in renal function. The abscess should be incised and **pus** and **blood sent for culture**. The most likely organism is *Staphylococcus aureus* and **intravenous flucloxacillin** is the drug of choice. However, until sensitivities are known, several antibiotics should be used. The acute tubular necrosis should resolve, and renal function return to its previous level. The chronic renal failure will, of course, need to be investigated in due course, but the most likely cause is chronic glomerulonephritis.

Because of his poor renal function, intravenous pyelography will not provide adequate visualization of his urinary tract, but **renal ultrasound scanning** will show renal size. Retrograde pyelography will rule out obstructive uropathy but this is most unlikely in this case. Further investigation would include **blood sugar, serum calcium and uric acid levels, serum proteins** and DNA **binding. Renal biopsy** would probably enable a firm diagnosis to be made, but could be delayed until the acute tubular necrosis had resolved.

Case 17

A 20-year-old American go-go dancer on holiday in London came to the casualty department with the following history. 24 hours before, her upper and lower lips had started to swell and on consultation with her GP antihistamines had been prescribed but to no avail. The swelling spread to involve the whole of the face and neck and was associated with tightness in her throat.

For the previous three years she had had intermittent localized swellings on her upper arms and lower legs which lasted two or three days. They were non-irritating and slightly pink in colour. Two years previously she had had a laparotomy for abdominal pain when an appendicitis was suspected but, at operation, a normal appendix was removed.

On examination she had gross non-pitting oedema of the face and neck. Both eyes were closed and the lips were very swollen. No rash was found. Examination of the cardiovascular, respiratory, alimentary and central nervous systems were normal. Urinalysis revealed no abnormality.

1. What further historical information would be helpful?
2. Suggest the most likely diagnosis and give one other possible diagnosis.
3. What was the cause of her abdominal pain two years before?
4. What is the immediate management of this patient?

The presentation is characteristic of **angioneurotic oedema** which presents with transitory episodes of localized oedema in subcutaneous and submucosal tissues. The disease may be **hereditary** (autosomal dominant) or **non-hereditary**. Thus, it is important to determine whether or not there is a **positive family history** (the mother of this girl died at the age of 27 following laryngeal oedema and respiratory obstruction). The hereditary form of the disease is often more severe and may manifest with **gastrointestinal obstruction** due to mucosal oedema. This is almost certainly the cause of the acute abdomen in this girl two years previously.

Hereditary angioneurotic oedema is associated in 85% of cases with a deficiency of C1 esterase inhibitor. The other 15% have normal levels of a clinically inactive inhibitor. Clinical attacks are attributed to the activation of C1, consumption of C2 and C4, and release of a vasoactive peptide. Attacks are often precipitated by trauma but may occur spontaneously.

Other conditions may present with oedematous swellings in various parts of the body, for example, **urticaria**. However, in these cases, which are manifestations of hypersensitivity phenomena, the lesions are accompanied by erythema and itching.

There are three aspects to treatment:

1. *The acute attack*. Although there is no definite evidence of benefit, most physicians would treat this with **adrenaline, antihistamines** and **steroids**. **Intubation** or tracheostomy may be required to preserve an airway.
2. *Short term prevention*. Before traumatic procedures, especially dental therapy, patients may be given two units of **fresh frozen plasma** as a source of C1 enterase inhibitor.
3. *Long term prophylaxis*. Antifibrinolytic agents such as ε-**aminocaproic acid (EACA)** have been shown to reduce the frequency of attacks and more recently the synthetic androgen **'Danazol'** has been proved highly effective with a lower incidence of side-effects. This would appear the treatment of choice, except possibly in pre-menopausal women. Local foci of infection that may precipitate attacks should be treated rapidly.

Case 18

A 68-year-old butcher was taken to casualty by ambulance from his niece's 21st birthday party with one hour of severe chest pain. Following an evening of celebrations he had become nauseated and went into the garden where he had vomited twice, bringing up altered food. He developed severe central chest tightness with sweating and continued to feel nauseated. He felt breathless. He had never previously experienced chest pains and had no relevant past medical history. He smoked 20 cigarettes daily and drank 20 pints of beer each week. He was allergic to penicillin which caused a rash.

On examination he smelt heavily of alcohol and was obviously in severe pain, clutching his anterior chest and moaning aloud. His pulse rate was 110/min, regular, BP 170/110 mmHg, venous pressure not raised, heart sounds normal and chest clear. He was afebrile and abdominal examination was unremarkable with no peritonism.

Investigations: ECG on arrival at casualty and repeated 1 hour later showed sinus tachycardia. Erect chest X-ray showed normal heart size, clear lung fields, no pneumothorax and no air under the diaphragm. Full blood count, urea and electrolytes, glucose, amylase and arterial blood gases on air all normal.

1. What is the diagnosis?
2. What further specific features would you look for in the above investigations?
3. What are the possible consequences?
4. What is the treatment?

This man developed severe chest pain after a bout of vomiting. There is no ECG evidence of acute myocardial infarction, although further ECGs should be carried out as should serial cardiac enzymes. There is no evidence of a pneumothorax, and pulmonary embolism is made less likely by normal arterial blood gases, although a ventilation–perfusion lung scan may be considered if all other causes are excluded. Acute pancreatitis or an intra-abdominal visceral perforation are less likely on the basis of investigations, but intrathoracic perforation is not excluded. The diagnosis is **oesophageal perforation (Boerhaave's syndrome)** following vomiting. This condition may also occur following oesophageal instrumentation during gastroscopy.

The chest X-ray may show a pneumomediastinum, mediastinal widening and a pleural effusion, often small and on the left side. The oesophageal perforation may be demonstrated by endoscopy or barium swallow. The possible consequences include:

1. Spontaneous closure of the perforation and resolution of symptoms.
2. Chemical pneumonitis, pneumonia or empyema.
3. Mediastinitis.

Although some advocate a conservative approach to management, most consider this condition a surgical emergency; increasing pain especially on swallowing, fever and evidence of mediastinal widening or pleural effusion are indications for an early surgical approach, with drainage, closure of the perforation and broad-spectrum antibiotics. The aim is to prevent mediastinitis which can be fulminant and fatal.

Case 19

A 20-year-old boy presented with transient episodes of left-sided weakness of his arm and leg which had come on over several weeks and appeared to vary in intensity. In the previous ten days he had two epileptiform seizures. He developed diabetes at the age of three and was now taking Actrapid insulin 32 units and Ultratard insulin 32 units daily. This dosage had recently been increased because of persistent glycosuria. He had noticed that he was hungry and eating more than usual.

On examination he was pale and sweating. All the abnormal physical signs were confined to the nervous system where the relevant findings were: cranial nerves normal; weakness of the left arm and left leg; increased reflexes in the left arm and leg with a left extensor Babinski response; increased tone in the left arm and leg; no sensory deficit.

Initial investigations in outpatients that afternoon showed: urinalysis 1% glycosuria, negative protein and ketones; Hb 13.5 g/dl; ESR 30 mm/h; blood sugar 4.5 mmol/l.

1. What four further investigations would you undertake?
2. Give four possible diagnoses.

This young man has a pure upper motor neurone lesion affecting his left side which is intermittent and has been associated with two fits. The combination of fits and his left-sided signs suggest that he has a progressive structural lesion involving his right cerebral motor cortex. The intermittent nature of these episodes suggests a possible fluctuating metabolic cause. He has had his diabetes mellitus controlled with reference to his urinary glucose. However, in outpatients he has a blood sugar of 4.5 mmol/l (80 mg%) with glycosuria, suggesting that he has a low renal threshold. **Hypoglycaemia** perhaps brought about by his recent increased insulin dosage, can produce transient neurological signs such as these; in particular, it can cause epilepsy, and his sweating on presentation may well be a clue to this diagnosis. Other likely explanations are that he has an expanding space-occupying lesion in his right motor cortex; he is diabetic and thus prone to infections, and a **cerebral abscess** is a diagnosis to be considered seriously, especially with the fits. Other structural possibilities are a **meningioma** or **glioma** or a **vascular malformation**.

Investigations must include **serial blood sugars** throughout the day and night to exclude hypoglycaemia. **Skull X-ray** may show a shift of a calcified pineal body or the calcification in an arteriovenous malformation. An **electroencephalogram** may show a localized focus with a space-occupying lesion or a more generalized disturbance in hypoglycaemia. **Enhanced computerized axial tomography** will show most localized structural lesions. CSF may be needed if no cause has been found to exclude infection. **Carotid arteriography** or **digital subtraction angiography** may be required if a space-occupying lesion is demonstrated and can show the abnormal blood supply of a tumour and stretching and displacement of arteries and localization of a mass in the case of other space-occupying lesions.

Case 20

A 54-year-old vicar was referred to the medical registrar in casualty. He had presented with a one-hour history of mild central chest tightness, palpitations, apprehension and sweating. Four years previously he had suffered an anterior myocardial infarction complicated by ventricular fibrillation and pericarditis but had not suffered post-infarction angina or heart failure, and was not followed up in hospital. The chest pain on this occasion was of similar quality but far less severe than that associated with his previous infarction. His GP had commenced him on disopyramide 100 mg twice daily six months previously for episodes of rapid, regular palpitations associated with dizziness occuring once a month and lasting up to two hours, although the episodes continued with the same frequency and he was awaiting an appointment to see a cardiologist. He did not smoke or drink alcohol, and took no other medications.

On examination he was alert and rational but was anxious. He was sweating with warm hands and feet, but he was afebrile and clinically euthyroid. Pulse rate 180/min and regular, blood pressure 120/80 mmHg with no paradox. Apical impulse impalpable. The venous pressure was not raised, and there were no obvious cardiac murmurs. The chest was clear and abdominal and neurological examinations normal.

ECG: regular tachycardia, ventricular rate 180/ min. QRS duration was 0.18 s, left bundle branch block pattern, no obvious P-waves. Chest X-ray, urea and electrolytes, full blood count and glucose all normal.

1. What are the two most likely underlying diagnoses?
2. Suggest the two likeliest causes of his current problem.
3. Describe four features including one therapeutic measure that may help to distinguish between these.
4. Suggest four further useful investigations.

This man has a history of previous myocardial infarction and recurrent palpitations. He is taking only a small dose of disopyramide. ECG shows a broad complex tachycardia. His original anterior myocardial infarction was complicated by ventricular fibrillation and acute pericarditis; these increase the likelihood of a **ventricular aneurysm** which may provide an arrhythmogenic focus. He may alternatively have an **ischaemic cardiomyopathy**. In the context of coronary artery disease and possible further myocardial ischaemia or infarction, he is most likely now to have **ventricular tachycardia. (VT)**. VT can occur with normal conscious level and without haemodynamic collapse. The alternative diagnosis is a **supraventricular tachycardia with bundle branch block (SVT with 'aberrant conduction')**. Aberration may be rate-dependent, or due to a conduction defect due to left ventricular disease from previous infarction. He is young for idiopathic conducting tissue disease.

In VT one may clinically detect beat-to-beat variation in pulse pressure, venous pressure (with canon waves) and in the first heart sound. ECG features which suggest VT include: AV dissociation, as evidenced by independant P-wave and QRS activity; fusion and capture beats; very broad QRS (> 0.14 sec); concordance (same polarity) of QRS complexes in all chest leads, V1–V6; deep S wave in V6; bifid QRS in V1 with a taller first peak (RSR pattern).

If there is haemodynamic collapse with cardiac arrest, heart failure, hypotension or diminished conscious level, treatment is with urgent DC cardioversion. In this particular case, one may try to restore sinus rhythm medically. Vagal manoeuvres may cardiovert an SVT but will have no effect upon VT.

Intravenous **adenosine** should be given. This naturally-occuring purine is becoming widely available and is useful for the treatment of SVT. It causes transient AV nodal block and terminates $> 80\%$ of SVT but has no effect upon VT. It is therefore also useful diagnostically. Adenosine is a benign drug and has no negatively inotropic effect, unlike verapamil which should **not** be given to this man as it may cause collapse. Whenever there is doubt, the rhythm should be assumed to be VT. If these measures fail and spontaneous cardioversion does not occur, elective DC cardioversion should be carried out. Investivations to consider include **serial cardiac enzymes** and **ECGs**, **echocardiogram** to assess ventricular function and look for LV aneurysm, **coronary angiography, ventriculography,** and **electrophysiological studies**.

Case 21

A 60-year-old widow came to outpatients and gave a clear history of four transient attacks of loss of vision in her left eye over the previous two weeks which she described 'like a curtain coming down over her eye'. The attacks lasted between five and ten minutes and the vision returned completely after the attack. One attack had been associated with some speech difficulty because a friend had not been able to understand what she said, but she had not noticed anything else wrong. Ten years previously she had had a peptic ulcer for which she had eventually required an abdominal operation. She was otherwise completely well and very fit for her age.

Her blood pressure was 190/110 mmHg, pulse 80 per minute, regular and of normal character. Significant findings were mild cardiomegaly and a systolic ejection murmur along the left sternal edge. There were no arterial bruits and ophthalmic and neurological examination were normal apart from an equivocal right plantar response.

Investigations showed Hb 12.7 g/dl, WBC 6.3 × 10⁹/1, ESR 22 mm/h. Chest X-ray normal, ECG: sinus rhythm, electrical left ventricular hypertrophy. Urine testing normal.

1. What would you look for in her fundi?
2. What would be your management and why?
3. What are the two most probable causes of her symptoms?
4. What would be the four definitive investigations?
5. What treatment is available?

This woman suffers from amaurosis fugax of her left eye, but the episode of dysarthria and the equivocal right plantar response suggest she had also suffered some cerebral ischaemia. The cause of her symptoms is likely to be recurrent emboli to the left opthalmic and middle cerebral arteries either from an atheromatous plaque in the **left carotid artery**, or else from a **cardiac lesion** and, if one dilates her pupils and examines the fundi carefully, one might find **cholesterol emboli** lodged in the arterial tree. Platelet emboli can sometimes be observed in the retinal arteries during an episode of amaurosis fugax.

The suggestion of cerebral ischaemia is most significant and this patient should be **admitted to hospital,** as she is at a substantial risk of developing a major CVA in the near future.

A cardiac source for the emboli should be excluded by **cardiac enzymes** and **echocardiography**. Fragments of a calcific aortic valve can embolize occasionally and these are seen in the retinal arteries as glistening pearly white fragments, quite different from cholesterol emboli. 24 hour tape monitoring would be necessary if one suspects an arrhythmia. **Carotid angiography** will define atheromatous plaques which usually lie at the bifurcation of the common carotid and do not always produce a bruit. Whilst these plaques can be removed by carotid endarterectomy, the feasibility of this depends on the general state of the patient. Most surgeons will require bilateral carotid angiography preoperatively and as this carries some morbidity in the elderly, it is only indicated if surgery is contemplated. **Doppler ultrasound** of carotid arteries is available in some centres and can provide non-invasive assessment of carotid lesions.

Antiplatelet drugs (in particular, **aspirin**) help to prevent further emboli from an atheromatous plaque, but one must be careful in view of the previous peptic ulceration. Anticoagulation does not have any beneficial effect on carotid atheroma, but is necessary if the patient has cardiac thrombus formation. Carotid endarterectomy has been shown to be associated with reduced mortality and morbidity as compared with medical therapy only in patients with bilateral severe carotid artery stenoses.

Case 22

An 18-year-old Moroccan girl, who had arrived in England three months previously, came to the casualty department with a month's history of sweats, intermittent fever, weight loss and lassitude. During this time she had had intermittent lower abdominal pain and heavy periods. Three days before admission she developed a painful rash on her legs. She had taken only aspirin for the fever during this time. There was no relevant past medical history.

On examination she was pyrexial (38°C) and thin. She had raised, hot, circumscribed nodules, 3 cm to 5 cm in diameter, which were tender, on her shins, forearms and lower trunk. All other systems were normal, except that on vaginal examination she was tender in the right fornix.

1. What is the skin rash?
2. What is the most likely diagnosis?
3. Give two other possible diagnoses.
4. Give six important investigations.

This young woman has **erythema nodosum** which may affect parts of the body other than the shins. She comes from Morocco and so **tuberculosis** must be high on the list of possible causes. Her only other physical sign is that she is tender on vaginal examination on the right. This, with her history of lower abdominal pain and menorrhagia, suggests pathology in her ovarian tubes or uterus. **Unilateral salpingitis** can be caused by tuberculosis and is the most likely diagnosis. **Crohn's disease** may also present with abdominal pain and may be associated with erythema nodosum. **Polyarteritis nodosa** can rarely also produce similar cutaneous lesions and is associated with pathology in the bowel. Other causes of erythema nodosum, such as sarcoid, ulcerative colitis and drug ingestion are not borne out by the history and clinical findings.

Investigations should be primarily orientated to excluding tuberculous salpingitis and should include **chest X-ray** and **ZN staining and culture for tuberculosis** of **sputum**, **urine**, and **high vaginal swab**. A **diagnostic dilatation and curettage** may provide bacteriological or histological evidence of turberculosis in the endometrium. A barium meal and follow-through is indicated if Crohn's disease is suspected, and investigations for polyarteritis nodosa should include anti-nuclear factor, hepatitis B antigen and appropriate biopsies.

Case 23

A 52-year-old bank clerk was referred with a six-week history of diarrhoea. She was opening her bowels up to 10 times daily, and passing watery, mucus-stained motions. She had some colicky lower abdominal pain but no vomiting, and her appetite was only slightly reduced; she had been drinking large quantities of fluids including Dioralyte electrolyte solution. Her husband was well, and they had not been abroad since a trip to Portugal two years previously. Her menopause had occurred at the age of 49 and she was experiencing occasional frontal headaches and hot flushes. Two weeks into this illness, her GP had commenced her on oral amoxycillin, but discontinued this due to a widespread pruritic maculopapular eruption. She was now taking only hormone replacement therapy. She had stopped smoking and drinking alcohol three months previously as these were making her feel unwell.

On examination, she looked well and was afebrile. She had clearly lost some weight. She was not jaundiced and had no lymphadenopathy. Pulse 96 regular, BP 150/70 mmHg, venous pressure not raised. There was a quiet ejection systolic murmur and an early diastolic murmur at the upper left sternal edge, louder on inspiration. Chest examination was normal. Abdominal examination revealed 3 cm firm, non-tender hepatomegaly, with no splenomegaly. There was no abdominal tenderness. Rectal and vaginal examinations were normal, as was sigmoidoscopy to 25 cm.

The following investigations were all normal: full blood count and film, urea and electrolytes, thyroid function tests, calcium, random glucose, amylase, chest and plain abdominal X-rays, barium enema to the caecum and ECG. Microscopy and culture of blood, stool and urine was normal, as was histology of two rectal biopsies taken at the time of sigmoidoscopy. Faecal mass 1200 g/24 h and faecal fat 0.3 g/24 h.

1. What is the diagnosis? Suggest two other possibilities.
2. Suggest six further important investigations.
3. What is the treatment?

This patient has diarrhoea of six-weeks duration. Bacterial infection with 'common pathogens' such as *Shigella* or *Salmonella* is unlikely, as these are usually self-resolving within this time period. However, further fresh stool should be sent for culture and for examination for ova, cysts and parasites. *Clostridium difficile* toxin should be looked for, although the sigmoidoscopic and biopsy features suggest neither pseudomembranous colitis nor ulcerative colitis. The barium enema is normal. The normal calcium, MCV, and low faecal fat excretion exclude steatorrhoea and significant malabsorption, making less likely but not excluding small bowel pathology such as Crohn's, giardiasis or lymphoma, and chronic pancreatitis. Further investigations include **small bowel follow through, jejunal biopsy** (with *Giardia* smear) and **pancreatic function tests, liver function tests** including **clotting screen** and **hepatitis** serology. This patient needs an **abdominal ultrasound** (particularly **liver** and pancreas) and possibly **abdominal CT scan.** If an abnormality is found in the liver, **liver biopsy** may be needed. A **gut hormone series** is needed, and **urinary 5-hydroxyindoleacetic acid (5-HIAA)**, the breakdown product of 5-HT should be measured. **Echocardiography** will help to define exactly the cause of her murmurs.

This woman has watery diarrhoea, pulmonary stenosis and regurgitation, flushing episodes despite hormone replacement therapy and firm hepatomegaly. These features gave the diagnosis of **carcinoid syndrome**; a primary tumour was found in the appendix with multiple hepatic metastases. Right-sided cardiac lesions include tricuspid regurgitation and occur in 50% of cases. Bronchospasm also occurs and flushing is often provoked by alcohol. The features are due to release of 5-HT and kinins. Treatment has been revolutionized by **octreotide,** an octapeptide analogue of somatostatin, which given subcutaneously inhibits gut hormone secretion and controls flushing and diarrhoea. Treatment may also include 5-HT antagonists, such as cyproheptadine, and surgical enucleation or selective embolization of hepatic secondaries if single or few in number; the latter may result in massive release of 5-HT and 'carcinoid crisis'. Chemotherapy with 5-fluorouracil is used in extensive disease. Median survival of patients with carcinoid tumours is 5–8 years, and 38 months for those with metastases and the carcinoid syndrome.

Case 24

A middle-aged male was brought into casualty unconscious. There were no accompanying relatives and he had been found in the local park.

On examination, his temperature was 37.8°C, blood pressure 90/70 mmHg, pulse 130 per minute, regular. His chest was clear and his abdomen was normal. Examination of his central nervous system showed that he was unresponsive to painful stimuli. His respiration was 14 per minute. His pupils were dilated, barely reacting to light. There was no meningism, tone was increased in all limbs and there were bilateral extensor plantars. The fundi were normal, and there were symmetrically brisk reflexes. General examination was unremarkable.

Investigations showed the following: Hb 13.0 g/dl, WBC 13 × 10⁹/l, platelets normal. Urea and electrolytes: sodium 131 mmol/l, potassium 4.0 mmol/l, urea 6.7 mmol/l. Blood sugar 4.8 mmol/l, calcium 2.32 mmol/l. Chest X-ray showed apical fibrosis in the right lung. Skull X-ray was normal.

Examination of the CSF showed: two lymphocytes. No red cells. Gram stain negative. Protein 0.4 g/l, sugar 3.8 mmol/l. OP 14 cm CSF.

ECG showed sinus tachycardia with occasional unifocal ventricular ectopics.

Shortly after the lumbar puncture he had two grand mal fits.

1. What is the diagnosis?
2. How would you confirm it?

The patient presents with a common clinical problem: a disordered state of consciousness and no available history. There are several possibilities including a post ictal state, cerebrovascular accidents including subarachnoid haemorrhage, infection either generalized or localized to the central nervous system, poor cerebral perfusion secondary to cardiac disease and, probably most common, drug overdose.

The commoner metabolic abnormalities are excluded by a normal glucose, calcium, urea and serum electrolytes. There is no evidence of meningitis and the mild leucocytosis in the peripheral blood is very non-specific and could have occurred following an unrecognized fit. Certainly for tuberculous meningitis to have caused such a disturbance of consciousness, the CSF would show some abnormality, even if AAFB were not seen.

The neurological signs do not localize any lesion and the findings of brisk reflexes, hypertonia and dilated pupils point to a generalized disturbance. In association with a sinus tachycardia and ventricular ectopics and the development of fits, a diagnosis of **tricyclic antidepressant overdose** is most likely. The severe overdose may in fact present with status epilepticus in which case the diagnosis may be delayed. The diagnosis is confirmed by **identification of the tricyclic compound** in **plasma**.

Treatment is supportive, with maintenance of an adequate airway and if necessary, intubation if respiration is significantly depressed. Gastric lavage and activated charcoal can reduce absorption but the airway *must* be protected by an endotracheal tube. Forced diuresis has no place in management. The treatment of arrhythmias is difficult, as most of the commoner anti-arrhythmics potentiate the cardiotoxicity of the drug. Generally, the arrhythmias in this condition appear to be fairly benign and do not need treatment. Occasionally, pacing and DC shock may be required. Coma may be reversed with the cholinesterase inhibitor, physostigmine, but it is short-acting and may precipitate convulsions and bradycardia.

Case 25

A 68-year-old publican presented with a one-month history of anorexia, malaise and a productive cough. The latter symptom was of a week's duration, the sputum being purulent with flecks of blood.

The patient had a partial gastrectomy for a duodenal ulcer ten years ago, but the operation was only partially successful and the patient's dyspepsia often required antacids. Four years ago he had had an inferior myocardial infarction but made a good recovery.

He drank four pints of beer per day and, until his infarct, smoked 25 cigarettes a day.

On examination, he was obese. His blood pressure was 150/90 mmHg, pulse 88 per minute and regular. He had normal heart sounds with an atrial gallop. In the chest, the percussion note was decreased at the right base, where there were coarse inspiratory crepitations. The abdomen was normal.

Investigations: Hb 11.6 g/dl, WBC 9 × 10⁹/l, platelets 286 × 10⁹/l, ESR 100 mm/h. Sodium 128 mmol/l, potassium 3.9 mmol/l, urea 4.2 mmol/l, bicarbonate 25 mmol/l, aspartate transaminase 36 U/l, alkaline phosphatase 112 U/l, bilirubin 16 μmol/l, total protein 91 g/l, albumin 28 g/l, calcium 2.70 mmol/l, phosphate 1.2 mmol/l, blood sugar 6.4 mmol/l, cholesterol and triglycerides normal. Serum osmolality 282 mosm/kg, urinary osmolality 512 mosm/kg.

Chest X-ray showed right basal shadowing. Sputum culture grew *Haemophilus influenzae*.

1. What is the most likely diagnosis?
2. Give five useful investigations.

This man presents with a non-specific history and a chest infection, for which there is almost certainly an underlying cause. In addition, he is mildly anaemic with a high ESR. The albumin is low and his globulins raised. He is hypercalcaemic, which is partly masked by hypoalbuminaemia and his phosphate and alkaline phosphatase are normal. This makes hyperparathyroidism and bony metastases unlikely. His hyponatraemia is not compatible with inappropriate ADH secretion, as there is no discrepancy between his serum osmolality (which is normal) and urine. In fact, he has a pseudohyponatraemia with a normal sodium concentration relative to a normal plasma water. However, in hyperlipidaemic or hyperproteinaemic states, the normal method for assaying sodium and calculating osmolarity are invalidated. In view of his normal lipids and a raised total serum protein, hyperglobulinaemia seems likely. Taken with the hypercalcaemia, **multiple myeloma** is the likeliest diagnosis.

Investigations should include **immunoglobulins, plasma protein electrophoresis, skeletal survey**, examination of the **urine** for **Bence-Jones protein and bone marrow biopsy.**

His chest infection, which cleared with antibiotics, could have caused hyponatraemia, as could a bronchial carcinoma. Hypercalcaemia due to milk alkali syndrome is accompanied by an alkalosis.

Case 26

A 43-year-old university lecturer was referred to medical outpatients because of recurrent headaches. These tended to occur at any time of the day, were throbbing in nature, situated at the vertex and frontal regions and lasted for between five minutes and an hour. The attacks had started four months previously and initially had occurred at three or four week intervals; however in the past month the attacks had occurred every four or five days. The headaches did not respond to aspirin, but the patient often experienced central abdominal pain and nausea during an attack and sometimes sweating. There were no visual symptoms either before or during an attack and there were no sensory symptoms in the limbs. He was on no regular medication and there was no significant past medical history.

Examination revealed a fit-looking man. Blood pressure was 130/90 mmHg supine and 95/60 mmHg standing; pulse 78 beats per minute and regular. There were no abnormalities in the heart, chest or abdomen. Examination of the central nervous system showed normal power, tone and sensation in all limbs. All reflexes were brisk and equal and both plantar responses were flexor. The cranial nerves were normal. Fundoscopy showed a small flame-shaped haemorrhage in the inferior temporal quadrant of the left eye and some arterial irregularity. There was no evidence of papilloedema.

Investigations showed: Hb 15.8 g/dl, WBC 8.4 × 10^9/l, ESR 40 mm/h. Urea and electrolytes, liver function tests and serum calcium were normal. Random blood sugar was 12.8 mmol/1. VDRL was negative; MSU was sterile. The chest and skull X-rays were normal, as was the contrast-enhanced CT brain scan. Barium meal and follow through showed no abnormality. Intravenous pyelography suggested flattening of the upper calyx of the left kidney. The upper pole of both kidneys was opposite the upper border of the 12th thoracic vertebrae. The ureter and bladder outlined normally.

1. What is the diagnosis?
2. How would you confirm this?

Headache is a common presenting symptom and the causes include the common 'tension' headache, migraine, temporal arteritis and causes of raised intracranial pressure due to a tumour. The clinical features of this patient's headaches are not particularly characteristic of any of these and in addition he has gastrointestinal symptoms and sweating. He is normotensive and on no medication, yet he has a degree of orthostatic hypotension. He also has mild diabetes and this could account for the haemorrhage in his left eye. Another possibility, however, is that he has had paroxysmal attacks of severe hypertension causing his headaches, which with the hyperhidrosis, suggests a diagnosis of **phaeochromocytoma**. The abdominal pain is a frequent symptom in paroxysmal episodes and may be due to bowel ischaemia—similar symptoms are seen in other states of increased adrenergic activity, e.g. clonidine withdrawal. Paroxysmal hypertension occurs in 40–50% of patients with phaeochromocytoma and the patient may be hypotensive following an acute episode (which often causes further delay in diagnosis). An alternative explanation for orthostatic hypotension is reduced plasma volume; however, recent studies have failed to confirm this finding in most patients with phaeochromocytoma.

Because the left kidney is normally higher than the right, the appearances on pyelography are suggestive of a suprarenal mass compressing the left kidney. There is now no place for potentially dangerous provocative tests (e.g. intravenous histamine) and diagnostic reduction of blood pressure with phentolamine has resulted in deaths from precipitous hypotension. **Urinary vanillyl mandelic acid (VMA)** and **metanephrines** are widely accepted as screening procedures, although false positives and false negatives are commonly found. **Plasma catecholamine** levels are almost invariably raised, but the patient should be resting and preferably not on vasodilator drugs, to avoid a spurious increase in plasma catecholamine levels. Multiple tumours occur in 10% of adults and a search for these should be made. Localization of tumours with flush aortography and renal arteriography, vena caval sampling, CT scanning—or adrenal MRI scanning—should be performed. Careful chest screening may exclude posterior mediastinal tumours. Scanning with radio-iodine labelled metaiodobenzylguanidine (^{131}I-MIBG) produces uptake in sites of excess catecholamine synthesis (chromaffin tissue)

Careful preoperative preparation, skilful anaesthesia and an experienced surgeon are vital for the surgical removal of the tumour.

Case 27

A 45-year-old carpet salesman was brought to casualty by ambulance. He had been unwell for three months, with non-productive cough, breathlessness and weight loss of 10 kg. His wife was convinced that the illness began after a dental extraction. He had received courses of amoxycillin and erythromycin from his general practitioner but the situation had not improved. On the day of admission he became much more breathless and agitated, and turned blue before suffering a generalized tonic–clonic seizure which lasted five minutes. He had no history of epilepsy, smoked twenty cigarettes a day and drank ten pints of beer each week.

On examination he was deeply unconscious with a Glasgow coma score of 3 and was centrally cyanosed. He had a coarse flapping tremor. The pupils were dilated and showed sluggish constriction to light, and the fundi were normal. The neck was rigid. Although afebrile, the peripheries were warm and he was sweating profusely. His tone was flaccid and there were no long tract signs; reflexes normal and plantars downgoing. There were no rashes. He was self-ventilating with a respiratory rate of 30 / min. Pulse 110 regular, blood pressure 190/115 mmHg. The venous pressure was not raised, heart sounds normal. Chest examination was unremarkable except for a harsh inspiratory and expiratory wheeze heard over the trachea but not over the lung fields. He was not jaundiced and there was no lymphadenopathy.

Investigations: glucose 8.7 mmol/l, Hb 12.3 g/dl, WBC 10 × 10⁹/l, platelets 504 × 10⁹/l, clotting screen normal, sodium 137 mmol/l, potassium 3.9 mmol/l, urea 3.9 mmol/l, corrected calcium 2.4 mmol/l, amylase normal. Arterial blood gases on air: PO_2 4.7 kPa (35 mmHg), PCO_2 17.2 kPa (129 mmHg), pH 7.01, bicarbonate 35 mmol/l, base excess: + 12. Chest X-ray showed no obvious abnormality. ECG showed sinus tachycardia with incomplete right bundle branch block. Urine and blood drug screen negative.

A procedure was carried out in casualty which resulted in a full recovery of consciousness within ten minutes.

1. What is the likeliest underlying diagnosis and give an investigation to confirm it?
2. What was the cause of the unconsciousness?
3. What procedure was carried out?

The history of breathlessness, cough and weight loss in a smoker should always raise the possibility of **carcinoma of the bronchus**. The seizure, followed by deep unconsciousness with dilated pupils and meningism may suggest an intracranial catastrophe such as a cerebrovascular accident or subarachnoid haemorrhage, or may be related to cerebral metastases. Meningitis or encephalitis are possibilities. None of these conditions, however, are associated with rapid recovery in consciousness following a procedure in casualty. There are no localizing neurological signs and a metabolic cause for unconsciousness should be considered. The long preceding history of breathlessness with sudden worsening, 'turning blue' before a generalized seizure and the features of meningism, dilated pupils, flapping tremor, warm peripheries and hypertension, together with wheeze over the trachea are consistent with **acute upper airways obstruction**. This is confirmed by marked hypercapnia and hypoxaemia, and the unconsciousness was due to **carbon dioxide narcosis**. If long-standing, papilloedema may occur. Obstruction of large airways is more often seen in children, following inhalation of a foreign body such as a peanut, and in anaesthetic practice, but it can occur as an unusual presentation of carcinoma of the bronchus, as in this case. The history of dental extraction was not relevant and no tooth was seen on chest X-ray! Laryngeal carcinoma may present in a similar way although a hoarse voice would usually be present. The diagnosis would be confirmed by **bronchoscopy** and **bronchial biopsy**. In this case, a fungating bronchial carcinoma was seen at the carina causing intermittent tracheal obstruction by a 'ball-valve effect'.

The procedure was **endotracheal intubation**.

Case 28

A 14-year-old girl presented to her local GP having felt unwell for ten days during which time she had a fever, developed a transient rash on her trunk and subsequently developed pain and tenderness in her left knee. He referred her to hospital where she was admitted.

On examination, her temperature was 38.5°C. She had non-tender cervical lymphadenopathy. Her blood pressure was 120/80 mmHg, JVP not raised, pulse 110 per minute regular, the heart sounds were normal and her chest was clear. In her abdomen her splenic tip was palpable. Her left knee was swollen, tender and hot.

Initial investigations showed: Hb 12 g/dl, WBC 13 × 10^9/l, ESR 90 mm/h, urine microscopy showed no protein or cells. Paul–Bunnell test negative.

Over the next four days she developed a swinging fever, painful wrists and pain in the neck on movement. On the fourth day she was found to have a pericardial friction rub but no murmurs and no evidence of cardiac failure. She later developed a red and painful left eye.

1. What would have been the three most likely diagnoses on admission?
2. What three important diagnostic investigations should have been carried out on admission?
3. With her subsequent course in mind, give the two most likely diagnoses.
4. How might her skin rash have helped establish the diagnosis?

The initial presentation with fever, pain and swelling of the left knee and a short prodromal history makes it imperative to rule out **infective arthritis** or **osteomyelitis** and **joint aspiration** with microscopy and culture of the aspirate must be performed. **Blood cultures** must be taken. Sometimes **acute leukaemia** will simulate a pyogenic arthritis, and a **peripheral blood film** was made on admission. Her subsequent course suggests a systemic disease. Rubella may be associated with arthritis, a history of rash and the presence of cervical lymphadenopathy, but it is not associated with pericarditis. The important differential diagnoses lie between **rheumatic fever, Still's disease, systemic lupus erythematosus** and **rheumatoid arthritis**. She is in the right age group for Still's disease and rheumatic fever, while young for SLE. The differentiation of rheumatic fever and Still's disease may be difficult as both have prodromal rashes (typically **erythema marginatum** or **maculopapular**), however, cervical spine involvement is more common in Still's disease, as is swinging pyrexia, lymphadenopathy and hepatosplenomegaly. A negative Paul–Bunnell test makes **infectious mononucleosis** unlikely.

Important investigations in this patient must include **serology for rheumatoid factor, anti-nuclear factor** and **DNA binding**, an **ECG** to assess cardiac involvement, **X-rays of involved joints** and a **chest X-ray**. A **full blood count** and **ESR, throat swab** and an **ASO titre** should also be performed.

It is important to examine the eyes of patients with suspected Still's disease with a slit-lamp to pick up iritis as this can be a serious complication and lead to blindness. The treatment of Still's disease includes bed rest as long as systemic symptoms are present, maintenance of good alignment of joints with splints and physiotherapy to maintain muscle function. Aspirin should be given for symptomatic relief.

Case 29

A 64-year-old businessman went to see his general practitioner accompanied
by his wife. She stated that she had become increasingly worried about her
husband who was often drowsy during the daytime and whose previously
successful business was beginning to founder. The man denied these
difficulties but did state that he had had difficulty in sleeping recently and
that his ankles had become swollen. He had previously been well except for
a hospital admission five years ago with a small, uncomplicated myocardial
infarction. He admitted to smoking five cigars per day and to drinking at
business lunches with an additional whisky as a night-cap.

The family doctor advised him to take a holiday and prescribed nitrazepam
at night for his insomnia, frusemide for his swollen ankles and Feospan as a
general tonic, as he thought the man looked pale.

A month later the man was brought into casualty having been very confused
and aggressive that morning. He had apparently initially improved following
his medication but more recently his ankle oedema had returned and he
had increased his diuretic therapy himself. In the three days before
admission he had become increasingly confused and drowsy.

On examination, he looked pale and had bilateral Dupuytren's contractures.
His abdomen was distended with dullness in both flanks and there was
bruising on both legs. Rectal examination revealed a black stool.
Neurologically, the man was stuporose, being rousable by pain, muscle
tone increased, his tendon reflexes all symmetrically exaggerated and both
plantar responses extensor. No sensory loss could be found.

Initial investigations showed: Hb 13.4 g/dl, MCV 104 fl, WBC 12 × 10⁹/l,
salicylate and paracetamol screens negative, glucose 4.7 mmol/l, sodium
132 mmol/l, potassium 2.9 mmol/l, urea 2.0 mmol/l. Chest and skull X-rays
normal. ECG showed an old inferior myocardial infarction.

1. What is the likely diagnosis?
2. Name five factors that may have caused his deterioration.
3. Name eight important principles in management.

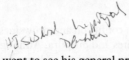

This man presents with confusion and drowsiness and on examination there is evidence of ascites and purpura. Although disseminated malignancy with abdominal and intracerebral secondaries could give a similar picture, his raised MCV and Dupuytren's contractures point towards an alcoholic aetiology. Patients often do not tell their true alcohol consumption. His neurological state is consistent with **hepatic encephalopathy** which can be of insidious onset. The most characteristic (but not diagnostic) sign the casualty officer should elicit would be asterixis (or flapping tremor). In anyone with neurological deterioration who might have been falling (bruises), it is important to exclude a subdural haematoma with a CT brain scan.

Deterioration of this man's encephalopathy may be due to:

1. A recent alcoholic binge.
2. Gastrointestinal haemorrhage—his black stool may be due to his iron therapy, but he might also have melaena.
3. Electrolyte imbalance (hypokalaemia or hyponatraemia) due to his frusemide.
4. His nitrazepam treatment–people in encephalopathy have increased susceptibility to sedatives.
5. Infection, which should be avidly looked for–especially septicaemia and infected ascites.

His management must include:

1. The avoidance of sedation, if at all possible.
2. Correction of electrolyte imbalance.
3. Curtainment of dietary protein.
4. Oral neomycin to reduce the colonic bacterial content.
5. Vitamin K, if necessary, to attempt to correct clotting abnormalities.
6. Treatment of infection or gastrointestinal haemorrhage, if applicable.
7. Cimetidine is useful to help prevent gastrointestinal haemorrhage.
8. Purgatives.

Case 30

A 30-year-old insurance broker felt unwell and lost his appetite on returning from a three week holiday in India. He developed flatulence and abdominal discomfort after food with, a few days later, diarrhoea. Four weeks later he went to see his doctor as his symptoms were continuing and he had lost a stone and a half in weight. He described his stools as pale and offensive. There was nothing of note in his past medical history.

On examination he was thin and pale. His abdomen was slightly distended although liver, spleen and kidneys were not palpable. His bowel sounds were increased. On rectal examination soft, shiny grey faeces were found and no abnormal masses were palpable. Sigmoidoscopy was normal.

Investigations: Hb 9.0 g/dl; urea and electrolytes normal; glucose tolerance test showed a flat curve; chest X-ray normal; barium meal and follow through showed a slightly dilated small bowel with coarse mucosal folds and some flocculation of the barium; 24 hour faecal fat 31.5 mmol/24 h (9 g/24 h); culture of faeces for *Salmonella*, *Shigella* and *Campylobacter* negative.

1. Name three likely diagnoses.
2. What further investigations would you perform to differentiate these?

This man has malabsorption, steatorrhoea and anaemia associated with four-weeks ill health after his return from India. His sigmoidoscopy was normal and his barium follow through showed changes compatible with his malabsorption with no other structural lesion. Infestations with protozoa and helminths are not uncommonly acquired in this geographical area and the most likely causing this picture would be **giardiasis**. This often causes an acute episode of diarrhoea which may merge into a chronic picture. It may be associated with a malabsorption syndrome although the aetiological significance of the Giardia has not been proven. Other parasitic infections that may cause steatorrhoea include strongyloidiasis and capillariasis (usually contracted in the Philippines). Ancylostomiasis (hookworm) may cause rapid and severe iron deficiency anaemia, but rarely malabsorption. The two other important differential diagnoses are **tropical sprue** and **adult coeliac disease**. With tropical sprue the visit abroad need only be brief and may be sometime before the onset of symptoms. Less likely causes, in view of the lack of specific radiological features, would be Crohn's disease, lymphoma or intestinal tuberculosis and rare causes of malabsorption are Whipple's disease and some collagen disorders. The abnormal glucose absorption makes liver, biliary or pancreatic disease unlikely.

Examination of the faeces for parasites is mandatory in this case. A **full blood count** and **film, serum iron and iron binding capacity** and **serum B12** and **red cell folate** should be performed. If parasites are not isolated from his faeces then a **small intestinal biopsy** should be performed. At the same time, **duodenal fluid** should be **aspirated** for parasites and these should also be sought on an imprint of the mucosal biopsy on a slide. The histological differentiation of coeliac disease and tropical sprue may be very difficult.

Even when giardiasis has been diagnosed it should not be accepted as the sole cause of malabsorption. The response to treatment, usually metronidazole, should be closely followed and further investigations performed if necessary.

Case 31

A 46-year-old man presented with a two-month history of progressive burning pains in the soles of both feet, especially the right, with cramps and shooting pains in both calves. His right leg had also become progressively weaker, and he had developed footdrop. Seven months previously he had been admitted to another hospital with fever, cough and pleuritic chest pains. He had been told that his chest X-ray showed a patchy shadow, and after a lung scan took warfarin therapy for six months. His general health had not improved and he had intermittent fevers. He had a history of asthma since the age of 35, for which he was receiving inhaled salbutamol and becotide, and of recurrent sinusitis. He had undergone a nasal polypectomy two years previously. He smoked ten cigarettes daily and drank five pints of beer each week. He had not travelled abroad.

On examination he looked well. He had no rash or lymphadenopathy. Temperature 37.4°C, BP 130/90 mmHg, pulse 96 regular, respiratory rate 18/min. There were some inspiratory and expiratory wheezes bilaterally, peak flow rate was 390 l/min. There was evidence of a bilateral sensorimotor neuropathy affecting both legs, with reduced sensation in response to pinprick, light touch, and temperature in the medial aspect of the right thigh and both feet, and reduced vibration and joint position sensation in both ankles. Dorsiflexion of the right foot was weak; further neurological examination, the heart and abdomen were normal.

Investigations: Hb 12.1 g/dl, WBC 22.5 × 10⁹/l, neutrophils 47%, lymphocytes 11%, eosinophils 39%, basophils 3%, platelets 407 × 10⁹/l. Urea 9.6 mmol/l, creatinine 155 μmol/l, sodium 139 mmol/l, potassium 4.2 mmol/l, glucose 4.8 mmol/l. Liver function and thyroid function tests normal. ESR 55 mm/h. Antinuclear and anti-DNA antibodies negative, rheumatoid factor negative. Syphilis serology negative, B12 and folate normal. ECG normal. Chest X-ray showed hyperexpansion with normal heart size. There were linear opacities with apical thickening in both upper lobes. There was a small patchy opacity at the left base. Mantoux negative at 1000 tuberculin units. Blood cultures sterile, urine normal. X-rays of the spine were normal, as was a CT and magnetic resonance (MRI) scan of the spinal cord and brain.

1. What is the most likely diagnosis?
2. Suggest three useful investigations.

This man presents with a multisystem disorder characterized by peripheral neuropathy, eosinophilia, low-grade fever, upper and lower respiratory tract symptoms and renal impairment. He has a history of nasal polyposis and sinusitis, and late-onset asthma. These features suggest a vasculitis, the most likely being **Churg–Strauss** syndrome. Wegener's granulomatosis may present in this way as may polyarteritis nodosa, although asthma and this degree of eosinophilia make Churg–Strauss likelier. Other causes of eosinophilia include parasitic infections, hypereosinophilic syndromes (e.g. Loeffler's), drugs, atopic diseases, haematological disorders and granulomatoses such as sarcoidosis.

Churg–Strauss syndrome is diagnosed clinically upon the presence of four or more of the following criteria (American College of Rheumatology, 1990):

1. Asthma.
2. Peripheral blood eosinophilia.
3. Neuropathy.
4. Pulmonary infiltrates.
5. Paranasal sinus involvement.
6. Biopsy showing vasculitis with extra-vascular involvement.

This approach allows discrimination from other vasculitides with a sensitivity of 85% and a specificity of over 99%.

Confirmation of the diagnosis is by **tissue biopsy**, such as **renal** or **nasal mucosal**. Histology may show heavy tissue infiltration by eosinophils, granuloma formation and/or a necrotizing vasculitis. The lesions are often dissociated temporally and spatially. Different organs have prediliction for different lesions: granulomatous nodules commonly occur in the heart and not the lungs, while nasal mucosa usually reveals only an eosinophilic infiltration without granulomas or vasculitis. Renal biopsy shows a focal, segmental necrotizing glomerulonephritis. **Anti-neutrophil cytoplasmic antibodies (ANCA)** are present in Churg–Strauss syndrome, and are of the p-ANCA type. Levels of **immunoglobulin E** are also elevated, although the possible role of either ANCA or IgE in pathogenesis is unclear.

The mainstay of treatment is with high-dose corticosteroids; in severe, rapidly progressive disease, pulsed methylprednisolone is given. Response is monitored by serial eosinophil, ESR and C-reactive protein estimations. Some patients require immunosuppression with cyclophosphamide or azathioprine.

Case 32

As the medical registrar on duty on the weekend you are asked by the obstetrics registrar to advise about the further investigation of a woman of 32 who is in the 14th week of her third pregnancy. Her first two pregnancies were apparently uneventful, but took place in Central Africa where she was unsupervised; all the children have the same father. She has felt extremely well throughout this pregnancy.

He tells you that she has been admitted with a blood pressure of 160/110 mmHg. She has a pulse rate of 100/min of normal character and regular. The obstetrics registrar has heard an ejection click in the aortic area and an ejection systolic murmur throughout the praecordium and back. He thinks that the rest of the examination is unremarkable and the ECG is normal. She has not had a chest X-ray. You agree to see the patient.

1. Using the information available so far, suggest the two diagnoses which together could link the findings in this woman.
2. What further specific feature of the examination do you wish to know?
3. Suggest the two most useful investigations.

Although incomplete, the information given can allow one to have some preliminary thoughts regarding the diagnosis. This young woman has hypertension, an ejection systolic murmur in the praecordium and back and an aortic ejection click. 'Innocent' systolic aortic flow murmurs or internal mammary artery bruits occur in pregnancy, but this murmur is not innocent if it is associated with hypertension and a click. Recent evidence suggests that pre-eclampsia relates to paternal antigens, and is therefore unlikely to occur for the first time in the third pregnancy with the same father.

The murmur need not necessarily arise from the heart itself. A unifying diagnosis would be **coarctation of the aorta** with a **bicuspid aortic valve**, the commonest association of aortic coarctation, causing the ejection click.

The crucial feature on physical examination is the presence of **radio-femoral delay**. The blood pressure should be measured in both arms and legs. There may be palpable collateral arteries around the scapula, sometimes associated with a bruit.

The most useful investigation is **echocardiography** with **Doppler studies**. In experienced hands, this can demonstrate the coarctation and estimate the gradient across it. The aortic valve can be assessed, as can left ventricular wall thickness. Transoesophageal echocardiography may provide more information than transthoracic. **Magnetic resonance imaging (MRI)** will also reveal the coarctation as will **aortography** although the latter should not be carried out in a pregnant woman.

Case 33

The patient was a 16-year-old male who was admitted with the following history: for the previous six months he had complained of a generalized weakness to such an extent that he was unable to play football at school. He had no other symptoms until the day before admission, when he felt generally unwell and had vomited on one occasion.

On examination, he was noted to be small for his age (below the 3rd centile for height and weight), but sexual development was normal. The remainder of the examination was unremarkable. The blood pressure was 100/70 mmHg.

Investigations were as follows: Hb 14.0 g/dl, WBC 6.0 × 10⁹/l. Plasma sodium 135 mmol/l, potassium 2.3 mmol/l, bicarbonate 32 mmol/l, urea 5.3 mmol/l. Plasma renin activity 12 ng/ml/h (high). Urine sodium 69 mmol/24 h, potassium 29 mmol/24 h. Estimations of total body water and total exchangeable potassium were below normal. Plasma cortisols were normal.

1. What is the most likely diagnosis?
2. Give two other possible causes for the electrolyte abnormalities present in this case.
3. What further investigations would confirm your most likely diagnosis?
4. What treatment may reverse the electrolyte abnormalities present?

This boy has muscle weakness, a normal blood pressure, hypokalaemia, increased serum bicarbonate concentration, and raised plasma renin activity.

Hypokalaemia may be associated with gastrointestinal loss of potassium (e.g. repeated vomiting, diarrhoea or purgative abuse), renal loss of potassium, diuretic therapy or abuse, licorice ingestion or therapy with carbenoxolone, and hyperaldosteronism, primary or secondary. Other causes include anorexia nervosa, diabetes insipidus and pyelonephritis.

In this case the normal blood pressure and high renin exclude primary hyperaldosteronism and other causes of mineralocorticoid excess. The 'normal' renal potassium excretion in the face of a low plasma potassium suggests inappropriate loss of potassium by the kidneys, and abuse of diuretics, e.g. thiazides could produce this picture, with stimulation of the renin-angiotensin-aldosterone system. Ingestion of sodium-retaining agents, e.g. licorice, would not be associated with low total body water, nor of elevated plasma renin levels.

This clinical presentation is that of **Bartter's syndrome**. The underlying abnormality is an intrarenal defect in sodium metabolism characterized by a reduced renotubular reabsorption of sodium leading to an increased fraction of filtered sodium being presented to the distal nephron where potassium is secreted. Thus, a greater fraction than normal of sodium and potassium is excreted in the urine. There is an increase in the renal synthesis of prostaglandins and this may lead to the hyperreninaemia and hyperaldosteronism. Furthermore a hyporesponsiveness of blood vessels to the pressor effects of angiotensin II can be demonstrated in these patients; thus, despite high levels of renin, the blood pressure does not rise above normal.

The diagnosis may be supported by **renal biopsy** where hyperplasia of the juxtaglomerular apparatus is characteristically seen; **reduced pressor responses to infused angiotensin II**; and **increased urinary prostaglandin excretion**.

Reversal of the clinical, electrolyte and other biochemical abnormalities in this syndrome occurs rapidly after treatment with **prostaglandin synthesis inhibitors** e.g. indomethacin.

Case 34

A 47-year-old woman was admitted to hospital with a two-day history of pain in the chest radiating down both arms. The pain was brought on initially by carrying heavy shopping bags, and was associated with shortness of breath, sweating and palpitations. On one occasion she vomited a small volume of unremarkable fluid. Apart from generalized weakness she had no other symptoms.

26 years previously she had had 'pleurisy' and was hospitalized for a year. No further details were available for this illness. Ten years ago she was diagnosed as having myasthenia gravis. Routine investigations at this time revealed a small thymoma, but surgery was not undertaken and the patient had been adequately controlled with anticholinesterases until the present admission.

Examination at the time of admission revealed a myasthenic facies and a pyrexia of 37.5°C. There was no cyanosis. There was a tachycardia of 140 per minute, sinus rhythm, poor volume. The blood pressure was 90/60 mmHg, the JVP elevated to the angle of the jaw, and the apex beat was not palpable. The heart sounds were very faint, no murmurs were present. Chest expansion was moderately good. There was dullness to percussion at the left base with no added sounds. The liver was palpable 3 cm below the right costal margin and tender. Bulbar weakness and generalized weakness of the limbs was noted.

Investigations showed: Hb 11.9 g/dl, WBC 14 × 10⁹/1, ESR 115 mm/h. Urea and electrolytes normal. Chest X-ray showed a uniformly enlarged heart and left pleural effusion. ECG was of low voltage with a sinus tachycardia and depressed ST segments in all limb leads.

1. Give two possible causes for her recent deterioration.
2. How could her previous history account for the cardiac findings?
3. What six further investigations would be most useful?

The initial history of chest pain and dyspnoea brought on by exertion suggests ischaemic heart disease. The information given in the history taken in conjunction with the examination findings provide alternatives. A low cardiac output, grossly elevated venous pressure, an impalpable apex beat and low voltage ECG must suggest a **pericardial effusion**. Kussmaul's sign is not easily demonstrated with gross elevation of neck veins, but pulsus paradoxus may be present.

From the history it may be that the previous pleuritic illness was **tuberculous** and this suggests a possible cause for the subsequent effusions. However, a **thymoma** was noted ten years previously, and a significant number of tumours of this type undergo **malignant change**. They spread by direct infiltration and invade the pericardium.

Her recent deterioration could, therefore, be due either to **ischaemic heart disease**, or to the development of a **pericardial effusion**. Other complications of myasthenia should be considered, such as bronchopneumonia or aspiration pneumonia. These could hardly account for all the physical signs.

Other causes for the pericardial effusion would include collagen diseases, for example SLE, and malignancy (spread from carcinoma of bronchus or oesophagus). Myxoedema is also a rare cause of pericardial effusions.

Further investigations should include **cardiac enzymes, echocardiography** and a **Mantoux test. Sputum** and **gastric washings** should be obtained for **acid fast bacilli**, culture and cytology. A **thoracic CT scan** may show an invasive thymoma. Examination of blood and serum should include a **full blood count**, estimations of **anti-nuclear antibodies** and **rheumatoid factor**. Finally, **pericardial aspiration and biopsy** should be performed, perhaps as a preliminary to thoracotomy.

Case 35

A 37-year-old insurance salesman had been well until the age of 32 when he first noticed mild unsteadiness of gait and altered sensation in the left hand. Two years later a diagnosis of possible multiple sclerosis was made. Symptomatically his condition remained static for five years after which he reported further deterioration in gait, oscillopsia on downgaze, incoordination of both arms and altered sensation first in the left lower limb and then in the right lower limb.

On examination he was noted to have a low cervical hairline. Heel-toe walking was impaired. Romberg's test was positive. There was downbeating nystagmus, and wasting and fasciculation of the left side of the tongue. Both plantar responses were extensor. There was impairment of joint position sensation in the hands more than in the feet and the two point discrimination threshold was 9 mm in all digits of the left hand.

1. What is the localization of this lesion?
2. Give two differential diagnoses.
3. What radiological investigations are indicated?
4. What investigations might have helped to confirm or exclude a diagnosis of multiple sclerosis when he was 34?

The patient's history and signs are typical of an abnormality at the level of the foramen magnum. The diagnosis was an **Arnold–Chiari malformation** with associated **cerebellar ectopia** (i.e. herniation of the cerebellar tonsils through the foramen magnum). A low hairline is associated with this condition. **Syringomyelia with syringobulbia** alone could produce such a picture, as could **congenital platybasia** or **basilar invagination** (the latter sometimes secondary to **Paget's disease**). A tumour at the foramen magnum such as a **meningioma, neurofibroma** or **chordoma** would also be a possibility. Downbeating nystagmus which produces oscillopsia when the patient looks down to read or to go down stairs is classical of lesions at this site. The history and signs are not characteristic of multiple sclerosis.

Radiological investigations should include **plain skull X-rays** with views of the skull base, **cervical spine X-rays, myelography** with adequate visualization of the cerebellar tonsils and craniocervical junction. **Computerized axial tomographic scanning** of the posterior fossa and upper cervical cord will demonstrate medulla compression or a syrinx. The most effective investigation is **magnetic resonance imaging (MRI scan)**. Vertebral angiography may be necessary to define a tumour circulation if surgery is contemplated.

A diagnosis of multiple sclerosis should have been supported by CSF examination with **cytology** and **protein electrophoresis** for typical oligoclonal IgG bands. **Visual evoked** and **brainstem evoked responses** should also have been sought. MRI Scanning will show high signals associated with areas of demyelination.

The patient underwent surgical decompression of the foramen magnum. The ataxia of gait improved over the next two years, but the nystagmus and oscillopsia remained unaltered and were really quite disabling.

Case 36

A woman of 29, recently married, went to her GP complaining of shortness of breath which had occurred spasmodically over the previous six months. Her attacks of dyspnoea had been worse at night and had not occurred during her summer holiday in Majorca. On examination the GP could find no abnormality and considered the attacks to be 'functional' in origin. However they persisted, and on three occasions a relief doctor had been called to see her at night and had prescribed an inhaler which had relieved her symptoms. When she was referred to a casualty department two months later, in an acute attack, she was breathless, distressed and on auscultation of the chest widespread rhonchi were audible, most pronounced on expiration. She responded slowly and only after several doses of intravenous aminophylline had been given. On admission to the ward she was started on steroids.

1. Name five physical signs that would help you assess the gravity of her situation?
2. How would your answers to the first question affect your further management of this patient?
3. What factors would suggest an allergic aetiology to her condition?
4. How would this affect your subsequent management?

Although attacks of breathlessness may well be functional or hysterical in nature, such a diagnosis should be entertained only after eliminating all possible organic causes. The intermittent nature of the episodes and freedom from symptoms between attacks strongly suggests asthma. The diagnosis is indeed borne out by the findings on her subsequent presentation in casualty.

The danger signs in a patient with asthma include **tachycardia, cyanosis, dehydration, exhaustion, hypotension, pronounced pulsus paradoxus** and the **inability to expectorate tenacious sputum**.

If necessary, further assessment can be obtained by simple spirometry, the peak flow rate and by the arterial blood gases. Early in the asthmatic attack, hypoxia occurs and the resultant hyperventilation causes hypocapnia. As fatigue sets in, however, hypoventilation ensues and the $PaCO_2$ starts to rise. This is a severe sign and often heralds the need to initiate **intermittent positive pressure respiration**.

Dehydration necessitates **fluid replacement**, orally or intravenously, and treatment of the severe case otherwise consists of **high dose oxygen therapy** (if no chronic obstructive airways disease), **bronchodilators** given intravenously and by inhalation, and **corticosteroids**. Some physicians would routinely give a broad spectrum antibiotic to cover any possible bacterial infective component. If ventilation is undertaken, then bronchial lavage can be performed to remove sputum plugs, although its efficacy is unproven.

Evidence of an allergic aetiology should be sought from a past **history** (and possibly family history) of **atopic diseases**. Besides asthma, these include eczema, hay fever and allergic rhinitis. It is important to take a detailed history of the attacks with respect to any possible **allergens** (such as house dust mite or animal danders). Atopic individuals have **high levels of circulating IgE** and specific sensitivity can be shown by **skin tests**, **radioallergosorbent tests** (**RASTS**) and, in a few centres, bronchial challenge tests. Therapeutically, it is important to pin-point specific allergies for the **avoidance of allergens** and the fact that **disodium cromoglycate** is more likely to be effective. Desensitization, although often helpful in children, is of little benefit in adult asthmatics.

Case 37

A 75-year-old woman who had suffered with arthritis affecting her hands, elbows and knees for 15 years was sent to casualty by her GP with a fever and dysuria which had not resolved on oral trimethoprim. Over the previous six-month period she had suffered two chest infections and a further urinary tract infection, all slow to resolve. She had lost 10 kg in weight. She took regular oral ibuprofen, prescribed by her GP for arthritis; she had never taken steroids. She was teetotal and a nonsmoker. Her husband had died two years previously of carcinoma of the lung.

On examination she looked frail and unwell, with a pyrexia of 37.8°C. She had generalized light brown skin pigmentation. She had a symmetrical deforming arthropathy with spindling and ulnar deviation of the fingers. She had a tender nodule over the right elbow. Pulse rate was 100/minute, regular and BP 130/80 mmHg. Cardiovascular, respiratory and neurological examinations were unremarkable. She had 4 cm splenic enlargement but no hepatomegaly or lymphadenopathy.

Investigations: Hb 8.0 g/dl, MCV 80 fl, platelets 95 × 10⁹/l, WBC 1.2 × 10⁹/l, neutrophils 60%, lymphocytes 35%. Urea and electrolytes, glucose, liver function tests, thyroid function tests, ECG and chest X-ray normal. Blood cultures sterile. A midstream specimen of urine grew > 10⁵ *E. coli*/ml, sensitive to gentamicin.

1. What is the diagnosis? Suggest another possibility.
2. Suggest five further investigations.
3. Suggest six explanations for the full blood count result.
4. What is the management?

The combination of long-standing rheumatoid arthritis in an elderly patient with splenomegaly, pigmentation, neutropenia and recurrent infections suggests the diagnosis of **Felty's syndrome**. Lymphadenopathy, weight loss, vasculitic skin ulceration and features of hypersplenism such as pancytopenia also occur. Neutropenia is due not only to hypersplenism but to associated antineutrophil antibodies. HLA DRW 4 is present in 95% of cases (compared with 70% of all patients with rheumatoid and 30% of the general population). Felty's syndrome affects 5% of older patients with rheumatoid arthritis and the rheumatoid factor is invariably positive, as may be other autoantibodies such as anti-nuclear factor.

Other causes of splenomegaly and pancytopenia must be considered. These include myeloproliferative disorders such as **multiple myeloma**, lymphoproliferative disorders, amyloidosis and some infections.

Further investigations should include **rheumatoid factor** and **autoantibodies, plasma protein electrophoresis; immunoglobulin estimation, urinary Bence–Jones protein, blood film, Coombs' test, haptoglobins, Philadelphia chromosome** and **leucocyte alkaline phosphatase, B12, folate, iron and iron-binding capacity. Bone marrow aspiration** and **trephine biopsy** is needed to exclude malignant infiltration.

The full blood count is likely to have a multifactorial basis in chronic rheumatoid disease:

1. Hypersplenism—causing pancytopenia.
2. Anaemia of 'chronic disease'.
3. Gastrointestinal blood loss due to non-steroidal anti-inflammatory drugs.
4. Bone-marrow suppression by drugs (e.g. gold and in the past phenylbutazone).
5. B12 deficiency due to associated pernicious anaemia.
6. Antibody-mediated haemolysis, neutropenia and thrombocytopenia.

Management should include a **neutropenic regimen**, with 'reverse barrier' nursing, combination antibiotics with anti-Pseudomonas activity (e.g. gentamicin and piperacillin or ciprofloxacin), careful mouth and perineal hygiene including oral antifungal mouthwashes, and avoidance of uncooked vegetables and salads. **Leucocyte transfusions** are used in severely ill neutropenic patients but rarely in the context of Felty's. Long term, **splenectomy** does not always help.

Case 38

A 54-year-old man came home drunk one night, and fell downstairs. His wife left him there until the morning, when he awoke and complained of a bad pain in his back and inability to move his legs. His wife and a friend carried him to bed, where he remained until the next day. As his legs were still immobile, he was sent to hospital.

When he was examined the neurological signs in the legs were: absent reflexes including plantar reflexes, a flaccid paralysis of all movements, absent pain and temperature sensation, but normal touch, vibration and joint position sensation. The absence of pain and temperature sensation extended onto his trunk up to a level corresponding to the T11 dermatome. The bladder was distended and the upper edge was palpated at the level of the umbilicus. He had no control over micturition. General examination showed a regular pulse, rate 96/min. There was difficulty feeling the pulse in the left arm, but it was easy to find on the right. The blood pressure in the left arm was 90/60 mmHg and in the right arm it was 160/110 mmHg. The pulses in the right groin and leg were impalpable. There was blood in the urine on microscopy.

A medical registrar made a diagnosis of polyarteritis nodosa. Soon after the patient reached the ward he complained of an excruciating pain between the shoulder blades, and dropped dead. Resuscitation was unsuccessful, and at necropsy the registrar was proved wrong.

1. Explain the neurological signs.
2. Suggest the correct diagnosis.

The only neurological functions preserved below T11 are touch, vibration and joint position sensation. These run wholly or in part in the dorsal columns of the spinal cord, dorsal to all other spinal cord tracts and neurones—including those mediating other sensations, motor functions, and bladder control—hence all the neurological abnormalities can be explained by a single lesion involving the anterior half of the spinal cord at and below T11. The symptoms were sudden in onset, so a vascular event seems likely. The anterior half to two thirds of the cord is supplied by the anterior spinal artery, so the lesion could be an acute obstruction of the anterior spinal artery.

There is also complete or partial obstruction of arteries in the left arm and right leg, and this picture of scattered arterial obstructions led the registrar to diagnose polyarteritis nodosa. Microscopic haematuria is found in polyarteritis nodosa when there is intrarenal arterial involvement, so this supported the diagnosis. However, the vessels involved in polyarteritis nodosa are usually much smaller than the major limbs arteries, and arteritis involving arteries of large size is very rare and usually presents with gradual rather than acute obstructions: Takayasu's disease is an example. Pain occurred at the start and at the end of this illness, and was at one time very severe.

The correct diagnosis must be of a disease that can progress to sudden death over a few days, intermittently very painful, causing acute obstructions of major arteries to the extent that blood pressure in the two arms can be different. At postmortem, an **aortic dissecting aneurysm** was found, and is compatible with all these features: the dissection extended from the arch of the aorta near the left subclavian artery to the bifurcation of the aorta and down the right common iliac artery. Haematuria is seen with dissecting aneurysm if the renal arteries are involved, and sudden death follows aortic rupture (as in this case) or retrograde dissection back to the aortic ring and pericardium.

Case 39

A 40-year-old bus conductor was referred for investigation. He was well until three months before admission, when he developed a flu-like illness with myalgia, night sweats and a cough productive of a little yellow sputum. His general practitioner thought he had a viral pneumonia and treated him with a variety of antibiotics and cough linctuses. Four weeks later he developed recurrent episodes of central abdominal pain coming on after food and only partially relieved by antacids. He had never vomited, but on two occasions he had had diarrhoea with some fresh blood in the stool. There was no previous history of note, but he had noticed a recent weight loss of 10 lb.

On examination, he had a temperature of 37.8°C. His blood pressure was 160/90 mmHg, and pulse was 108 per minute. Chest examination showed inspiratory bilateral wheezing. The abdomen was normal, but on sigmoidoscopy he had second degree piles. General examination was otherwise unhelpful.

Investigations: Hb 11.4 g/dl, WBC 17 × 10⁹/l, platelets 380 × 10⁹/l, ESR 60 mm/h. Urea and electrolytes, chest X-ray and barium meal were all normal. Bilirubin 16 μmol/l, aspartate transaminase 83 U/l, alkaline phosphatase 140 U/l. Sputum culture was sterile. His ECG showed a sinus tachycardia.

1. What is the diagnosis?
2. How would you establish it? Give six other useful investigations.

This man has a generalized illness causing respiratory and abdominal symptoms. His yellow sputum was sterile and although this may have been due to antibiotic therapy, a search for **sputum eosinophils** should be made. This is particularly relevant in view of his bronchospasm. His abdominal pain is highly suggestive of mesenteric ischaemia and a **barium meal and follow-through** may show 'thumbprinting' of the small bowel due to mucosal oedema. It will also exclude a peptic ulcer and a neoplasm.

The presence of vascular disease and a high ESR suggests a vasculitis, which in a man of this age, suggests **polyarteritis nodosa**. A **differential full blood count** may show eosinophilia and neutrophilia and in combination with a high ESR is very suggestive. Blood should be examined for **hepatitis B surface antigen** in view of the abnormal liver function tests and is present in up to 30% of all cases. The absence of **anti-nuclear antibodies** will exclude systemic lupus erythematosus. Histological evidence of vasculitis with characteristic polymorph infiltrate and fibrinoid around arteries is characteristic. Favoured sites for biopsy are kidney, muscle, testicle or skin nodules. In this case, however, there are no skin lesions, and there are no definite indications for renal biopsy. Muscle biopsy has a low success rate and testicular biopsy, although recommended by some authorities, has yet to gain widespread acceptance. Arteriographic changes have been found to be helpful in the diagnosis of polyarteritis nodosa.

In this patient, **selective mesenteric angiography** is indicated—the finding of multiple aneurysms of the same and varying size in visceral arteries is almost pathognomonic.

In microscopic polyarteritis, presentation is usually with a nephritic syndrome with myalgia and purpura. **Anti-neutrophil antibodies (ANCA)** may be present in the serum.

Case 40

A 33-year-old policeman was referred to outpatients after his GP had found his blood pressure to be 170/115 mmHg at an insurance examination. Physical examination showed no abnormalities apart from tortuosity of the retinal vessels, and investigations revealed no underlying cause for his hypertension. Within four weeks his blood pressure returned to 140/90 mmHg on a diuretic.

He was next seen eight weeks later when the following story was obtained. Five days after the start of a mild flu-like illness, he had noticed slight numbness of the right side of his face, and two days after this he had experienced sudden vertigo and vomited twice. Three days later his vertigo had worsened and he became severely ataxic with a tendency to fall to the right. Over the following week he became unable to walk, and other symptoms included tinnitus and partial deafness on the left side.

On examination, apart from a blood pressure of 170/120 mmHg, abnormal findings were confined to the CNS. The fundi showed tortuosity of vessels with no papilloedema. There was bilateral nystagmus on both lateral and vertical gaze, an absent right corneal reflex and minimal right facial weakness with impaired hearing on the left. There was gross incoordination of the limbs with dysdiadokokinesis. All limb reflexes were brisk. Abdominal reflexes were absent and the plantar responses were equivocal.

1. Give three possible causes for his recent illness.
2. What three investigations are indicated?

Concerning this patient's recent neurological illness, the problem is to decide whether this illness is related to his hypertension or whether it is an unrelated condition.

Considering the former—the stepwise progression of the CNS signs is against a **brain stem haemorrhage** although a succession of small bleeds from a vascular malformation is a possibility. Multiple emboli could present in this way but there was no obvious source in this patient. **Thrombosis in the vertebrobasilar arterial system** would be likely in an older patient and several cases have been reported in younger patients with hypertension or diabetes.

In view of the history of a flu-like illness preceding the neurological episode, a **post viral demyelination** should be considered.

Less likely possibilities include a posterior fossa lesion and of these a **cerebellar haemangioblastoma** could account for both hypertension and neurological signs.

Investigations indicated include **computerized axial tomography** and **magnetic resonance imaging**, a **lumbar puncture** (with examination for cells, protein and immunoglobulin), and a **vertebral arteriogram**, or **digital subtraction angiography**.

The diagnosis in this patient was vertebrobasilar artery thrombosis. Apart from hypertension, no other precipitating factors for this early presentation of cerebrovascular disease were found in this patient. Four years later he presented with angina on effort and gross triple vessel atheromatous disease was found on coronary angiography.

Case 41

A 48-year-old woman had been working in an East African mission hospital for three years where she had looked after the physiotherapy and radiology departments where she had worked two afternoons a week. Following an attack of diarrhoea she went to her doctor and was found to have a Hb 8.2 g/dl, WBC 2.3 × 10⁹/l (70% lymphocytes), platelets 60 × 10⁹/l. There was no history of drug ingestion in any form. She was not on a contraceptive pill and did not take any malaria prophylaxis. Apart from being pale there were no other abnormal physical signs and a bone marrow biopsy showed a uniform decrease in all elements with fatty replacement; no abnormal cells were seen.

It was felt she should stop working in the radiology department. She continued to be pale and six months later returned to England where she was given unknown quantities of iron, folic acid and vitamin B12. One year after her return to England she was seen in outpatients where she was found to have Hb 6.2 g/dl, WBC 1.8 × 10⁹/l (lymphocytes 65%), platelets 60 × 10⁹/l. A splenic tip was palpable on careful examination but there was no hepatomegaly and no other abnormal signs. Two attempts at sternal marrow biopsy were unsuccessful.

1. What are the three most likely diagnoses?
2. What would be the four most useful investigations?
3. How would you monitor her progress?

The haematological investigations suggest that this patient is pancytopenic, and this may be due to **aplastic anaemia (bone marrow failure)** or to **bone marrow replacement**. **Hypersplenism** is a less likely cause. Splenomegaly makes an **idiopathic aplastic anaemia** unlikely. There is no history of exposure to drugs or toxic chemicals (e.g. benzene) and although **radiation** is a possible cause, one might expect it to have a more rapidly fatal course. **Paroxysmal nocturnal haemoglobinuria** may present in this way and a history of haemoglobinuria should be sought. Tuberculosis may cause a hypoplastic marrow but with this length of history one would expect more constitutional symptoms.

Investigations should include an **iliac crest trephine** and **aspiration**, a **blood film**, **Ham's test** for acid haemolysis and **urine examination** for haemoglobin and haemosiderin.

Aplastic anaemia tends to carry a poor prognosis due to infections and haemorrhage. Treatment lies in blood transfusions and attempts to stimulate the marrow with androgens such as oxymethalone, although proof of efficacy is lacking. The response to treatment is monitored by serial haemoglobin, reticulocyte and platelet counts. Some centres initiate intensive immunosuppressive therapy with significant response in up to 50% of patients in some series.

Bone marrow transplantation is available to some individuals who have an HLA-matched sibling donor.

Case 42

A 60-year-old man was referred to hospital for investigation of the following symptoms: for the past two years he had noticed progressive difficulty in passing urine and had become impotent. During the last three months he had felt dizzy when rising from his bed in the mornings and also occasionally during the day when getting up from a chair. On four such occasions he had lost consciousness for about one minute.

On physical examination he was noted to have a mild right-sided Parkinsonian tremor of the hand. Examination of the cardiovascular system revealed a regular pulse of 90 beats per minute and a recumbent blood pressure of 180/90 mmHg. There was no cardiomegaly and auscultation of the heart was normal. He was not in cardiac failure. Examination of the respiratory and alimentary systems was normal and the following abnormalities were found on examination of the nervous system: he had evidence of a pseudobulbar palsy and bilateral pyramidal signs on examination of the limbs. He had an ataxic gait and further testing showed evidence of bilateral cerebellar disturbance.

1. How may his history of loss of consciousness be related to the neurological disturbances?
2. What is the most likely diagnosis?
3. What further investigations would confirm your answers to questions 1 and 2?

The symptoms of dizziness and loss of consciousness on rising to the upright position are strongly suggestive of **orthostatic hypotension**. Such symptoms are commonly precipitated by drugs and may occur to some extent with advancing age. However, in this case, the history is strongly suggestive of more widespread autonomic impairment and the finding of abnormal pyramidal tract signs, cerebellar dysfunction and Parkinsonism, are all features of **multiple system atrophy (Shy–Drager syndrome)**.

Tests of autonomic function should include the **Valsalva manoeuvre** which in this case demonstrated an absence of any overshoot of blood pressure during Phase 4 of the manoeuvre. Also, the cardio-accelerator response (increase in pulse rate during Phase 2) was absent. The influence of carotid massage may show absence of slowing of the cardiac rate in autonomic dysfunction and the vasoconstrictor response to cold is also absent in many patients with efferent lesions of the sympathetic pathway.

Biochemical tests of noradrenaline release from sympathetic nerve endings into plasma usually reveal low–low normal levels of noradrenaline and a failure of the levels to rise with tilt is characteristic of autonomic failure.

Treatment of orthostatic hypotension is largely unsuccessful and has included mineralocorticoids, the use of pressor drugs and anti-gravity suits. Recent reports of benefit from beta-blocking drugs and prostaglandin synthesis inhibitors have not been confirmed in other studies.

Case 43

A 15-year-old West Indian boy had felt unwell for four days with myalgia, lethargy, vague central abdominal pain and vomiting. Several days later his ankle became tender and he was admitted to hospital. His past medical history contained no similar episodes, but he had had recurrent sore throats.

On examination, his temperature was 38°C, his throat was inflamed, but there was no pus visible. Blood pressure was 115/70 mmHg; pulse rate 100 beats per minute. Examination of the cardiovascular system, chest and central nervous system was normal. Examination of the joints revealed mild swelling of the right elbow and tenderness over the right knee. Abdominal examination showed some tenderness around the umbilicus, but no peritonism. Rectal examination was normal, except that the stool was positive when tested for blood. General examination was normal, apart from a mildly inflamed pharynx.

Investigations: Hb 14.3 g/dl, WBC 7.4 × 10⁹/l (normal differential). Platelets 340 × 10⁹/l. The blood film was normal and the Paul–Bunnell test negative. Chest X-ray and urea and electrolytes were normal. Blood and urine cultures were sterile. ESR was 30 mm/h.

His abdominal pain resolved over the next week on conservative management, but routine urine testing two weeks after his admission showed haematuria. The urine was sterile on culture.

1. What is the most likely diagnosis?
2. What disease could present with an identical clinical picture?

A combination of swollen joints, abdominal pain with blood in the stools and haematuria suggests a diagnosis of **Henoch–Schönlein purpura**, a condition in which circulating immune complexes produce widespread damage to vascular endothelium and vasculitis. A maculopapular rash is often, but not always, present, classically involving the ankles, buttocks and elbows. Other causes of polyarthralgia must be considered, including juvenile rheumatoid arthritis, rheumatic fever (now rare) and the arthritis associated with ulcerative colitis and Crohn's Disease. Serum sickness is most unlikely without a recent history of immunization or drug ingestion. Infectious mononucleosis is unlikely in view of the normal blood film and negative Paul–Bunnell test. However, other viral infections, e.g. rubella and mumps, can present with an acute polyarthritis. Acute leukaemia is unlikely with a normal blood picture and 'collagen diseases' are rare in this age group. Abdominal pain, joint symptoms and haematuria may all occur in a **sickle-cell crisis**. The lack of previous episodes and a normal haemoglobin makes this unlikely, however, and the normal blood film and absence of sickle cells excludes the diagnosis.

In **Henoch–Schönlein purpura** severe complications may result from vasculitis affecting the gut and may lead to haemorrhage, perforation, or intussusception. The renal lesion may vary from a mild focal nephritis (usually presenting as slight or intermittent haematuria) to more severe acute glomerulonephritis with diffuse hypercellularity and crescents (proteinuria and progressive impairment of renal function). The prognosis is worse in adults and this is mainly due to the severity of the renal lesion.

The disease usually settles in 4–6 weeks, without sequelae, but may be recurrent.

Case 44

A 30-year-old radio reporter attended casualty with a two-day history of breathlessness at rest. Following a sore throat two weeks previously, he had developed a cough occasionally productive of small blood clots. He had no chest pain. He was usually in excellent health. His wife and 5-year-old son had also had sore throats but both had recovered fully without breathlessness. He smoked 30 cigarettes daily and drank five pints of beer each week.

On examination he looked well, but was centrally cyanosed and became breathless while undressing and when talking. His temperature was 37.4°C and pulse rate 100/min, regular. Blood pressure 120/70 mmHg. No pulsus paradoxus. Examination of the chest revealed bilateral inspiratory and expiratory wheeze but was otherwise normal. Peak expiratory flow rate 550 l/min.

Investigations: Hb 9.8 g/dl, WBC 11 $\times$ 10^9/l, platelets 480 $\times$ 10^9/l, ESR 91 mm/h, urea 14 mmol/l, sodium 133 mmol/l, potassium 4.8 mmol /l, creatinine 162 μ mol/l. ECG showed sinus tachycardia, Chest X-ray showed widespread patchy interstitial shadowing in the left midzone and right mid- and lower zones with no cavitation and normal heart size. Arterial blood gases on air: PaO_2 7.8 kPa (59 mmHg), $PaCO_2$ 3.1 kPa (23 mmHg), pH 7.46.

A diagnosis of bronchopneumonia was made. He was commenced on oxygen and high doses of intravenous ampicillin, gentamicin and erythromycin. The morning after admission, he suffered a large haemoptysis and subsequently had a cardiac arrest. He was resuscitated, intubated and ventilated. A repeat chest X-ray showed dense opacification in the left mid- and lower zones and throughout the right lung field. Despite inotropic support he died 12 hours later.

1. What is the likeliest diagnosis? Suggest an alternative.
2. What is the treatment?

This unfortunate young man illustrates the important point that shadowing on a chest X-ray is not necessarily infective. Following a sore throat, he developed marked dyspnoea, hypoxaemia and haemoptysis. He had a low-grade fever, and the blood tests revealed anaemia, a normal white cell count, a high ESR and renal impairment. The chest X-ray showed widespread interstitial shadowing. He did not respond to broad spectrum antibiotics, suggesting either that his condition was non-infective or that the agent involved was not sensitive. **Goodpasture's syndrome** was the diagnosis at postmortem; intrapulmonary haemorrhage can produce this picture, although it is not always this dramatic. Patients often present with marked hypoxaemia and chest X-ray abnormalities but look quite well. A **viral pneumonia** is an alternative, usually associated with mild respiratory but severe systemic symptoms, and is frequently missed; a low neutrophil count and negative sputum and blood cultures would be expected, the diagnosis being made retrospectively on the basis of **rising antibody titres** or isolation of virus from **throat swabs**. *Legionella pneumophila*, *Mycoplasma pneumoniae* or an **ornithosis** should respond to intravenous erythromycin and like **tuberculosis** are rarely this dramatic.

Goodpasture's syndrome is one of pulmonary haemorrhage and glomerulonephritis. It typically affects young men who smoke, and sometimes follows a viral infection. Antibodies are present directed towards glomerular and alveolar basement membrane antigens; these **anti-basement membrane antibodies** can be measured. **Renal biopsy** shows glomerular immunoglobulin deposition in a linear pattern.

Treatment is with **plasmapheresis** which can dramatically improve the clinical situation, and with **immunosuppression** with agents such as corticosteroids and azathioprine. Renal failure is sometimes progressive and severe and may require **dialysis** or **transplantation** when anti-basement membrane antibodies have disappeared. Most patients recover.

Case 45

A 25-year-old woman with insulin dependent diabetes for 15 years was admitted to hospital in ketoacidotic coma. On recovery, she complained that the sight in both her eyes had been progressively deteriorating for the past six months.

Apart from the abnormalities in both eyes and proteinuria, the physical examination was normal.

1. What further investigations would you perform?
2. What are the three potential causes for her visual problems?

Her diabetes was subsequently controlled on twice daily Actrapid and Ultratard insulin.

3. What alteration in vision would you expect to follow such treatment?
4. What further therapy might be indicated to help her vision?

Progressive deterioration of vision in a young diabetic may result from a number of pathological conditions within the eye, of which the most serious is neovascularization of the retina (retinitis proliferans). The disease of the small blood vessels is, of course, not confined to the eyes and may involve the glomeruli and give rise to impaired renal function. This girl already has proteinuria and thus assessment of renal function with **creatinine clearance** and **24 hour protein excretion** should be performed and this will determine the long-term prognosis of the patient.

Visual failure in diabetes can result from **cataracts**, to which diabetics are more susceptible, or the retinopathy which causes visual loss either by producing **macular oedema** or a **proliferative retinopathy**. Background retinopathy does not cause visual loss. Young diabetics occasionally rapidly develop a 'snowflake' cataract, but premature 'senile' types of cataract are more commonly found. There is now good evidence that meticulous control of blood sugar is associated with a slower progression of retinopathy and patients should be encouraged to monitor their own blood sugars, possibly with home glucose meters. There is no doubt that panretinal photocoagulation with either laser or xenon light is of benefit to proliferative retinopathy, but photocoagulation of a maculopathy is of less certain benefit because, although the retinal changes can be reversed, visual improvement does not follow. However, some authorities argue that further deterioration is halted and that in future maculopathies may require much earlier treatment. Pituitary ablation or clofibrate no longer have any place in the treatment of retinopathy. Sophisticated vitreous surgery is increasingly successful in removing vitreous haemorrhages and replacing traction retinal detachments in the late stages of retinitis proliferans.

Following stabilization of her diabetes, there are osmotic changes in the lens which become **less myopic** and there will be changes in vision. This can take several weeks and spectacles should not be prescribed until the eyes have stabilized. Any remaining loss of visual acuity is likely to be due to lens changes and the retinopathy.

There is evidence that treatment with angiotensin converting enzyme (ACE) inhibitor drugs may reduce the rate of progression of diabetic retinopathy and nephropathy.

Case 46

A 37-year-old right-handed garage mechanic had become aware of impaired hearing in the left ear when aged 34. At the age of 36 his friends commented that he sometimes walked as though he had been drinking and he himself noted that his gait would become very unsteady after drinking a single pint of ale (much reducing his capacity for alcohol).

On examination his gait was unsteady and he tended to veer to the left. Romberg's test was positive. There was a coarse, large amplitude, poorly sustained, first degree nystagmus on left lateral gaze and a finer, smaller amplitude first degree nystagmus to the right. Facial sensation was normal, the right corneal reflex was brisk, the left diminished and there was some weakness of the left facial muscles. Hearing was normal on the right, but he was unable to hear a watch tick at 1 foot on the left. Weber's test (using a tuning fork at 512 Hz) was lateralized to the right. With Rinne's test: right AC > BC, left BC > AC. There was mild incoordination of the left upper and lower limbs. The left plantar response was flexor, the right extensor.

1. What is the site of the lesion?
2. Give at least two causes.
3. How do you explain the results of the tuning fork test?
4. What would you expect caloric tests to show?
5. What investigations are indicated?

The presentation is that of a **cerebello-pontine angle lesion**. Tumours arising at this site include a meningioma, dermoid, epidermoid, metastasis, angioma or glomus tumour. An intrinsic brainstem lesion such as a glioma is unlikely in the absence of other cranial nerve signs. The most likely diagnosis in this patient is a **left acoustic neuroma** extending extracanalicularly and into the posterior fossa. These usually arise from the inferior branch of the vestibular division of the VIIIth nerve and a common finding on caloric testing is an **ipsilateral canal paresis**.

Pure tone audiometry showed that the patient was completely deaf in the left ear. The Rinne test result is known as a **false positive** as on testing BC the patient actually hears the tuning fork with the opposite ear. The coarse nystagmus to the side of the lesion is a gaze paretic nystagmus indicating disruption of vestibulo-cerebellar connections, the fine nystagmus to the right is gaze evoked nystagmus indicating cross compression of the brainstem vestibular nuclei.

Investigations should include **plain skull X-rays** with views of the **internal auditory meati, audiometry, caloric testing** and **brainstem evoked potentials. CT (scan)** with contrast enhancement with views of the porus is necessary and **magnetic resonance imaging (MRI scan)** if available. **Vertebral angiography** is often necessary to define the tumour's vascular supply preoperatively. The patient should be examined for cutaneous evidence of neurofibromatosis.

Case 47

Benuti Syplus -
hopal curdulud

A 20-year-old girl student went to see her college doctor after returning from her Easter holiday. She had a three day history of fever, sweats, and muscle pain, and in the last 24 hours had developed ulceration of her tongue and mouth and a very sore throat.

Three weeks before this illness she had been in Turkey on holiday and had been prescribed pain killers by a local doctor. There was no past medical history of serious illness.

On examination she was pyrexial (38.5°C), sweaty and dehydrated. She had oral ulceration and enlarged lymph glands in her neck. The rest of the examination was normal.

Investigations showed a Hb of 13.0 g/dl, WBC 1.5 × 10⁹/l; platelets 200 × 10⁹/l, Paul–Bunnell was negative; bilirubin 6.8 μmol/l, aspartate transaminase 15 U/l, alkaline phosphatase 95 U/l.

1. What is the most likely diagnosis? Give one other possibility.
2. What investigations should be performed. Give five.

This woman has an acute illness associated with leukopenia. Her leukopenia is most likely to be due to neutropenia and only a few disease processes cause severe neutropenia giving rise to symptoms; there are, **drug-induced neutropenia, idiopathic chronic neutropenia, acute aleukaemic leukaemia** and **aplastic anaemia**. A drug-induced neutropenia would be the most common cause of this picture and she has been treated with an analgesic in Turkey. In that country, Amidopyrone, which has been banned in Great Britain, is used as an analgesic and is a well-recognized cause of agranulocytosis. Other drugs which may cause this could include thiouracils and phenylbutazone. Even in the absence of a palpable spleen and no fall in haemoglobin or platelet count, **acute leukaemia** must be considered. She does not have the history of a chronic infection, which is often the hallmark of idiopathic chronic neutropenia. Infectious mononucleosis can give this picture rarely, but she has a negative Paul–Bunnell and other unusual causes are viral infections such as influenza or atypical viral pneumonia or brucellosis, but the degree of neutropenia in these cases rarely cause symptoms.

Leukaemia has to be excluded and investigations should therefore include a **blood film** and **marrow examination**. **Blood cultures** should also be done to exclude an associated septicaemia. **Throat swabs** and **ulcer scrapings** are necessary to isolate pyogenic organisms and fungi from the lesions in her mouth.

Treatment must be aimed at the primary cause, secondary infection and the prevention of further infection. She must have bactericidal antibiotics, and she must be barrier-nursed. Any drug which could possibly cause this reaction should obviously be stopped. Leukocyte transfusions are sometimes used in the acute phase.

Case 48

A 33-year-old computer programmer went to see his GP with intermittent fever, malaise, myalgia and sore throat for one week. He also had a mild headache and arthralgias. He was normally well and on no medication. There was no known contact with infectious disease and no recent travel abroad.

On examination he looked well but was flushed with a pyrexia of 37.8°C. He had slightly enlarged tender cervical and right inguinal lymphadenopathy. He had a pharyngitis. The remainder of the examination was normal.

Investigations: Hb 13.5 g/dl, WBC 5.4 × 10⁹/l (55% neutrophils, 45% lymphocytes), platelets 160 × 10⁹/l, ESR 40 mm/h. Film showed some abnormal mature monocytes. Chest X-ray and liver function tests normal, Paul–Bunnell test negative. Blood and throat swab cultures negative, serology for CMV and Toxoplasma negative.

One week later the patient returned asking for a medical certificate for his employers. He now felt tired but otherwise asymptomatic, and his physical signs had resolved.

1. What is the most likely diagnosis?
2. What further investigation would you like?
3. Describe three other ways in which this condition may present.

This man presents with a two-week history of non-specific malaise, fevers and myalgias and is found to have enlarged lymph glands in the neck and groin and a pharyngitis. His investigations show a lymphocytosis and atypical monocytes on a blood film, which would point to a diagnosis of infectious mononucleosis. However, Paul–Bunnell test is negative making the diagnosis far less likely, although the appearance of heterophil antibody may be delayed. There are several other causes of a syndrome resembling infectious mononucleosis with a negative Paul–Bunnell test. The most common are due to infection by **cytomegalovirus** and *Toxoplasma Gondii*; serological tests for both these were negative. Viral hepatitis may present in this way although lymphadenopathy is usually less marked and the liver function tests are normal. Hep BsAg and anti-Hep A IgM should be checked. Bacterial causes such as **brucellosis, tuberculosis** and **infective endocarditis** should be considered but are not in keeping with the history or findings and would not resolve spontaneously this quickly; similar reasons make a **lymphoma** unlikely.

Acute seroconversion to **human immunodeficiency virus** (**HIV**) can present with a short-lived glandular fever-like illness of this sort, and the **anti-HIV antibody** test, carried out after appropriate counselling, was positive. Seroconversion occurs 6–12 weeks after contact, and is often not diagnosed, as it may be **asymptomatic**, or may present with a mild **flu-like illness** with non-specific features. Acute infection may also present with **encephalopathy, neuropathy, meningitis** or a **myelopathy**. Clinical recovery from the seroconversion illness is often complete within one or two weeks.

Case 49

malignancy [handwritten]   *Windsor* [handwritten]
campylon [handwritten]

A 35-year-old doctor returned from a two year trip to Central Africa where he and his wife have been helping to set up a new hospital. He was concerned that despite being back in the UK for three months he had continued to lose weight and still had watery diarrhoea which had troubled him and his companions intermittently throughout their time in Africa. He otherwise felt well and was now taking no medications; he took antimalarial prophylaxis erratically during his trip. He was a non-smoker and drank one bottle of wine each week. His wife was well.

anaemic [handwritten]

On examination he was thin but looked well and was suntanned. He had pale conjunctivae. There was no lymphadenopathy and he was not jaundiced. He had splenomegaly extending to the umbilicus. There was no other obvious abnormality.   *Brudkly, IM, cryoporold* [handwritten]

Investigations: Hb 8.4 g/dl, WBC 3.1 × 10⁹/l, normal differential, platelets 90 × 10⁹/l. Blood film showed fragmented red cells. Urea and electrolytes, liver and thyroid function tests, glucose and calcium normal. Thick blood film showed no malaria parasites on three occasions. Stool culture showed no growth of Salmonella, Shigella or Campylobacter. Chest X-ray and ECG were normal.

1. Suggest the two likeliest diagnoses.
2. Suggest four useful investigations.
3. Is the clinical detection of splenomegaly ever a 'normal finding'?

This man who has been in Africa has a long history of intermittent diarrhoea and fever and has massive splenomegaly with pancytopenia. An infective cause has to be considered and **visceral Leishmaniasis (kala-azar)** is highly likely. Patients often look remarkably well despite dramatically abnormal physical findings and investigations. Lymphadenopathy and a cough are other common features. **Leishman–Donovan bodies** may be demonstrated in blood buffy coat, bone-marrow smears or in splenic, hepatic or lymph node aspirates. **Anti-Leishmania antibodies** may be detected by ELISA or indirect immunofluorescence. Leishmania may be **cultured** in Nicolle–Novy–MacNeal medium. An intradermal **Leishmanin skin test** may be positive.

Malaria causing **tropical splenomegaly syndrome** is another likely diagnosis. Negative malaria films are compatible with this diagnosis; malarial parasites are in fact not detected in either blood or splenic tissue. Very high levels of circulating **immunoglobulin M (IgM)** are found. **IgM aggregates** are found by immunofluorescence within hepatic Kupffer cells. Antimalarial therapy leads to regression of splenomegaly. **Schistosomiasis, brucellosis** and **tuberculosis** can also cause splenomegaly although it is rarely massive. Investigations should nevertheless include **Brucella serology**, a **tuberculin test** and a search for **Schistosoma ova** in urine and stool or on rectal biopsy. Anti-Schistosoma antibodies can be measured. Human immunodeficiency virus (HIV) is not a recognized cause of massive splenomegaly.

Non-infective causes of massive splenomegaly include **myelofibrosis** and **chronic myeloid leukaemia**, and although the patient is a little young for these and the WBC is low, **bone marrow aspiration** and **trephine biopsy** and **Philadelphia chromosome** should be checked. A **lymphoma** is possible, and if other investigations are negative, a search for intrathoracic and intra-abdominal lymphadenopathy should be made, initially by **computerized tomography** and **magnetic resonance imaging**. A **splenic biopsy** may be necessary.

Clinical splenomegaly is never normal; it is only palpable if enlarged three-fold or more. A prospective study of soldiers during the Vietnam War showed all those with clinical splenomegaly to have existing or subsequent haematological disease.

Case 50

A 28-year-old teacher was admitted through casualty. He gave a one-week history of abdominal distention and bloody diarrhoea, fever and anorexia. In the three days leading to admission, he had become progressively more breathless and the day before admission developed headache and drowsiness. He took no medications and had no contact with similarly affected cases. He had not travelled abroad.

On examination, he looked unwell and was cyanosed. His respiratory rate was 28/min, pulse 120/min, BP 90/60 mmHg, temperature 38°C. His chest was clear to clinical examination and heart sounds were normal. There was abdominal distention with absent bowel sounds but no peritonism, and rectal examination showed watery blood-stained diarrhoea. Neurological examination revealed a man who was drowsy but rousable, disorientated, with no focal long-tract signs. No meningism or photophobia. Fundoscopy revealed cotton wool exudates and widespread bilateral perivascular sheath haemorrhages.

Investigations: abdominal X-ray showed gas-filled distended loops of small and large bowel. The chest X-ray revealed bilateral widespread fine interstital shadows, normal heart size. Hb 9.0 g/dl, WBC 2.8 × 10⁹/l (95% neutrophils) platelets 90 × 10⁹/l, ESR 100 mm/h. Clotting screen and urea and electrolytes normal. ECG: sinus tachycardia. Arterial blood gases on air: PO_2 6.0 kPa (45 mmHg), PCO_2 2.5 kPa (19 mmHg), pH 7.35. Stool microscopy showed red cells but no white cells. Stool culture negative for Salmonella, Shigella and Campylobacter. Urine culture and microsopy normal, blood culture sterile.

1. What is the most likely diagnosis?
2. Suggest four useful diagnostic tests.
3. What is the treatment?

This man presented with a history initially dominated by bloody diarrhoea and abdominal distention but he subsequently developed a syndrome comprising encephalitis, retinitis and pneumonitis in addition to colitis. He had a high ESR, and was anaemic, thrombocytopenic and leucopenic with a relative lymphopenia. The diagnosis which explains this presentation is systemic infection with **cytomegalovirus**. This is an 'opportunistic infection' which affects immununosuppressed individuals, particularly those with impaired cell-mediated immunity. After counselling, this patient was found to have a positive test for **anti-human immunodeficiency virus (HIV) antibodies**. Systemic CMV infection means that he has developed the **acquired immunodeficiency syndrome (AIDS)**. The **lymphocyte CD4: CD8 ratio** is low, and there is often a **polyclonal increase in immunoglobulin levels**. The picture would also have been in keeping with bone marrow failure, for example due to **leukaemic infiltration**, and a **bone marrow aspiration** and **trephine biopsy** would make that diagnosis. CMV infection could be diagnosed by demonstration of dense round intracellular inclusions ('Owl's eyes') within swollen cells following a **rectal biopsy**, or by elevated **anti-CMV IgM levels** in **blood** or **CSF**.

Diarrhoea is a common problem in individuals with chronic HIV infection. It may be due to a proctitis, colitis, upper gastrointestinal pathology or systemic illness. Proctitis is commonly 'non-specific', or due to viral infection (e.g. herpes simplex, Epstein–Barr) or to gonococcal, treponemal or chlamydial infection. Colitis is caused by the 'common' bacterial pathogens and also agents such as Entamoeba and Cryptosporidium; the cysts and oocytes respectively of these should be specifically looked for on stool microscopy. Upper GI causes of diarrhoea include Giardia, lymphoma or Kaposi's sarcoma.

Treatment is usually symptomatic but CMV can be treated with **Ganciclovir**, although this can cause further leucopenia and thrombocytopenia and is a potential carcinogen. This man should also receive long-term treatment with **zidovudine (AZT)** in the hope of slowing the progression of HIV infection and with **nebulized pentamidine** or **oral co-trimoxazole** to reduce the risk of *Pneumocystis pneumonia*.

CMV retinitis is the commonest cause of visual impairment in patients with AIDS and untreated can result in bilateral blindness.

Case 51

A 30-year-old man was brought into hospital in an emergency. His friends said that two years previously he had been treated for thyroid trouble with tablets but had not bothered to take these for several months, during which time he had become progressively less well, tired, irritable and short of breath. He smoked at least 30 cigarettes a day, and had stopped working two months previously. Two days before admission he had started to cough up blood and greenish sputum and his condition had deteriorated dramatically; he was now too short of breath to get out of bed.

On examination the man was febrile and obviously very ill. He was drowsy and when roused thought that 'the doctor was the devil come to bury him alive'. He was dirty and unkempt with a marked tremor of his hands and wasting of his body. There was a large pulsating goitre with a systolic thrill and bruit. The pulse was 210 per minute and irregular. His blood pressure was 90/60 mmHg and he had signs of marked cardiac failure and cyanosis. Both eyes were severely proptosed and chemotic but showed no corneal staining with fluorescein.

Whilst in hospital over the next week, he developed deterioration in visual acuity.

1. What drugs would you use to control immediately this man's thyroid state?
2. What other drugs and supportive measures are indicated?
3. Give two possible causes and their treatment for his deterioration in visual acuity.
4. What is the long-term treatment of choice?

This man is an uncontrolled thyrotoxic, now in a state of thyroid crisis probably precipitated by a chest infection. Thyroid crises carry a 20% mortality even with immediate and strenuous treatment.

The objectives of treatment in the short-term are to inhibit further synthesis of thyroid hormones and to antagonize their peripheral effects, to treat any underlying precipitating cause and generally to support the patient.

Further synthesis of thyroid hormones can be rapidly blocked by the administration of **iodide** (10 mg four hourly orally). **Carbimazole** (10 mg q.d.s.) should be used in combination as the effect of iodide is often lost after ten days. Treatment of peripheral thyroid hormone effects with propranolol should not be started until the heart failure has been controlled. His precipitating chest infection should be vigorously treated with **antibiotics** after obtaining sputum and blood for culture. Thyrotoxic cardiac failure with atrial fibrillation will respond slowly to **digoxin** and **diuretics** but marked improvement will start when thyroid hormones are lowered to normal. General supportive measures are very important; these patients are hyperpyrexial and require vigorous cooling and soluble **aspirin**. Dehydration is often a problem and intravenous fluids with calories may be needed. **Hydrocortisone** is often given, as corticosteroids suppress many of the manifestations of thyrotoxicosis.

Deteriorating vision could be explained either by the development of **exposure keratopathy** or proptosis causing traction ischaemia or compression of the optic nerve from muscle infiltration. The involvement of extraocular muscles usually produces diplopia rather than visual loss. Treatment for exposure keratopathy initially should include **methylcellulose eyedrops** and **guanethidine eyedrops** and **tarsorrhaphy** may well be required. Visual loss from proptosis is an indication for high dose corticosteroids and immunosuppressives, and if there is continued deterioration, surgical decompression of the orbit should be carried out. VERs are useful to monitor visual function.

The alternative long-term treatments in this patient are medical treatment, radioactive iodine or surgery. He is a fickle person, having already failed to take his medication and so the choice lies between thyroidectomy or a therapeutic dose of radioactive ^{131}I.

Case 52

A young woman of 25 presented to her GP with galactorrhoea which had been present for six months. One year ago she had been admitted to a mental hospital with a nervous breakdown and had remained in this establishment for three months. She had regular menstruation and was taking the oral contraceptive pill.

1. Give three possible diagnoses.
2. Give four important investigations.

This woman has galactorrhoea which is most probably associated with hyperprolactinaemia. A raised serum prolactin may be caused by a **prolactinoma** in the pituitary gland or brought about by **drug therapy** or associated with **myxoedema**. She has recently been in a mental institution where she may well have received phenothiazines, which can cause hyperprolactinaemia. She is also on the oral contraceptive pill, which is a recognized cause of hyperprolactinaemia and galactorrhoea. Most patients with hyperprolactinaemia have amenorrhoea, but she is on the oral contraceptive pill and having regular withdrawal bleeds.

Investigation must include the measurement of a **serum prolactin.** It is important to exclude a prolactinoma; these are usually microadenomata, but further investigation to exclude a pituitary fossa expanding lesion must include **lateral skull X-ray** and **pituitary tomography**, a **computerized axial tomographic scan** and assessment of **visual fields**. An **MRI scan** of the pituitary fossa may give further information. Her **thyroid function** should also be measured. If there is no evidence of a pituitary adenoma, a first step would be to take her off the oral contraceptive pill and also any other drugs which cause raised prolactin levels. If this did not bring about a drop in her prolactin level and a cessation of galactorrhoea, treatment with bromocryptine for a pituitary microadenoma should be considered. Visual field changes would be an indication for pituitary surgery (transsphenoidal) which would also have to be considered with an expanded pituitary fossa.

Case 53

A 72-year-old woman was admitted as an emergency after her family doctor had found her collapsed at home. He had been treating her for a virus infection for the previous six days, during which she had been feeling weak and lethargic with shortness of breath and a cough.

On examination she was semiconscious, confused and dehydrated. She had atrial fibrillation with an apex rate of 140 per minute, blood pressure 130/95 mmHg. There were no focal neurological signs.

Investigations showed: Hb 16 g/dl; WBC 12 × 10⁹/l, blood urea 16.6 mmol/l, plasma sodium 150 mmol/l, potassium 5.5 mmol/l, chloride 97 mmol/l, bicarbonate 22 mmol/l, blood sugar 65 mmol/l, urine sugar 2%.

1. What is the cause of this patient's collapse?
2. What five further investigations are indicated?
3. Suggest five important steps in treating this patient.

MSU   IVi   Osmolality
ABG   Fluid
ECG   Insulin
CXR.   Antibiotics
BC.   ABs

This patient has profound hyperglycaemia and dehydration, but is not acidotic. She therefore presents with **hyperosmolar, nonketotic diabetic coma**. This condition has a high mortality and is often associated with late onset diabetes or, alternatively, it may be the presenting feature of the disease. Characteristically, severe hyperglycaemia is associated with dehydration, hypernatraemia, and hyperosmolality of plasma. Although ketoacidosis is not usually found, hyperosmolality and ketoacidosis may co-exist. However, investigations should include **blood gases** to determine acid-base status. In this patient who presents with a cardiac arrhythmia, an **ECG, chest X-ray** and **cardiac enzymes** would be mandatory. Investigations for a precipitating underlying infection should be sought and should include **sputum, blood** and **MSU culture**.

Treatment of this type of diabetic coma requires **rehydration** and the administration of **insulin. Hypotonic (N/2) saline** is often used initially and **short-acting insulin by a constant infusion**, often with smaller doses than required for ketoacidotic states, will reverse the metabolic abnormality. Frequent estimation of **blood sugar** and **electrolytes** are essential and intravenous therapy and insulin infusion should be adjusted according to these results.

Digitalization for atrial fibrillation would also be indicated and **broad-spectrum antibiotics** should be started after obtaining the specimens for culture.

Hyperosmolar coma causes increased blood viscosity and prophylactic anticoagulation with **heparin** is advisable.

Case 54

Atypical, AAW-Oral? (handwritten)

A 27-year-old labourer was admitted to hospital with an acute right lower lobe pneumonia following an upper respiratory tract infection. Although sputum cultures were sterile (he had received two days treatment with tetracycline before admission), he responded well to benzyl pencillin. His fever settled within 24 hours of admission and his general condition improved. At this time, he was noted to have haematuria on routine urine testing, but urine culture was sterile. Microscopy confirmed haematuria, but there was no pyuria. However, when urine culture was repeated four days later, microscopy was normal with no cells or casts visible. He was discharged from hospital and one month later he was discharged from the outpatient clinic as his chest X-ray showed complete resolution of his pneumonia.

Berger's nephropathy. (handwritten)

Six months later he reattended the clinic with a six day history of haematuria following a flu-like illness, which had started one week earlier. There was no accompanying abdominal pain or dysuria. There was no other significant past medical history.

On examination, no abnormalities were found. His blood pressure was 120/75 mmHg.

The patient was admitted at once for investigation. Full blood count, urea and electrolytes, calcium, liver function tests and clotting screen were all normal. Chest X-ray and IVP showed no abnormality. MSU showed RBCs + +, but no casts and was sterile on culture. Cystoscopy was normal.

1. What is the diagnosis?
2. How would you confirm it?

This patient has had repeated episodes of confirmed haematuria. Cystoscopy and IVP are normal, so the most likely cause of painless haematuria in an otherwise well person is glomerulonephritis. The occurrence of haematuria in association with a febrile illness is very suggestive of **Berger's disease** (**IgA nephropathy**). It occurs almost always in young or adolescent boys, often associated with an upper respiratory tract infection. Haematuria occurs at the same time or shortly after the upper respiratory symptoms, and may last for several weeks. The haematuria that occurs with acute post-streptococcal glomerulonephritis may occur transiently at the beginning of the illness, but is at its height on about the tenth day. In recent years, post-streptococcal glomerulonephritis has become extremely rare in the United Kingdom. During an acute attack of Berger's Disease, there may be transient impairment of renal function, but there is no fluid retention and the patients remains normotensive. Some patients have persistent proteinuria with or without haematuria. The condition is often benign and transient, but when there are recurrent attacks, the prognosis is less good—up to 10% of patients will develop hypertension and chronic renal failure. Patients under 15 years of age tend to do much better than the older age group, even though they may have recurrent attacks.

The necessary investigation is **percutaneous renal biopsy** which would show a mild focal and segmental proliferative glomerulonephritis. In contrast with the patchy nephritis, IgA and C_3 are deposited in all the glomeruli.

Case 55

A 46-year-old man was referred to the outpatient department complaining of a dull aching pain in the right hypochondrium that had been present for the last two months. He had, however, been feeling generally weak and lethargic for the last year and had lost one stone in weight. On further questioning, he admitted to impotence for six months and said he had decreased his frequency of shaving over this time. He did not smoke and drank two pints of beer on a Saturday night. In his past medical history he had suffered from arthritis in both knees for the last five years but was otherwise well. His only medication was an occasional paracetamol for this arthritis.

On examination, he looked well, being sun-tanned after a recent holiday in Greece. He was not anaemic, jaundiced, cyanosed or clubbed and there was no lymphadenopathy. Pulse 84 per minute, regular with ectopics. JVP + 7 cm. Cardiac apex in the anterior axillary line. He had a prominent third heart sound but there were no murmurs. Chest clinically clear. In the abdomen, the liver was palpable 3 cm below the costal margin, smooth and firm, and the spleen could just be tipped. He had bilateral testicular atrophy and there was crepitus in both knees. Urinalysis negative.

1. What is the most likely diagnosis?
2. How would you confirm this?

This man presents with rather non-specific symptoms of lethargy, weight loss and an abdominal ache. In addition, however, he has signs of cardiac failure with a displaced apex beat, mildly raised venous pressure and a third heart sound. This, in the absence of any valvular lesion, would raise the possibility of a cardiomyopathy. He also has testicular atrophy and hepatosplenomegaly and these, with his heart disease, suggest the diagnosis of **haemochromatosis**. He may well also be pigmented, this being confused with or hidden by his sun-tan and, in addition, his arthritis might be related, perhaps through chondrocalcinosis. Although his urinalysis is negative, this does not exclude mild diabetes that should be looked for.

Secondary causes of haemochromatosis should be excluded. These include anaemia with ineffective erythropoiesis (e.g. sideroblastic anaemia), alcoholic cirrhosis and a high oral iron intake. These appear unlikely in this man who probably has **idiopathic haemochromatosis** and a positive family history should be looked for.

Diagnosis is confirmed biochemically and histologically. The **serum concentrations of iron and ferritin** are usually raised as is the **percentage saturation of transferrin**. The **desferrioxamine test** can be used to confirm the presence of parenchymal iron overload. The 24 hour urine secretion of iron is raised following intramuscular desferrioxamine. **Liver biopsy** is considered the most reliable criterion for the evaluation of both parenchymal iron overload and tissue damage. All first-degree relatives over the age of 10 years should be screened biochemically for iron overload. This should be repeated at regular intervals. In most families the disease is inherited as an autosomal recessive trait. The affected gene has been localized to chromosome 6.

MRI scanning of the liver for screening relatives shows early promise. Treatment is with venesection and iron-chelating agents. 30% of patients with cirrhosis develop hepatocellular carcinoma.

Case 56

A 57-year-old lorry driver was admitted at the request of his general practitioner. He was normally well apart from his usual morning cough and white sputum, which he attributed to smoking 30 cigarettes a day. Two days before admission his sputum had increased and turned green and he had become increasingly lethargic and breathless. He was on no medication and drank two pints of beer a day.

On examination, he was febrile, dyspnoeic and cyanosed but not clubbed. His tongue was dry. Pulse 130/min and regular; blood pressure 130/80 mmHg. Auscultation of his chest revealed an area of bronchial breathing together with a few crackles at the left base. He had a fine tremor, his reflexes were brisk and there were no focal neurological signs.

Investigations: Hb 14.2 g/dl, WBC 24 × 10^9/l (95% neutrophils), ESR 70 mm/h, sodium 132 mmol/l, potassium 3.6 mmol/l, urea 4.0 mmol/l, glucose 5.0 mmol/l. Aspartate transaminase 30 U/l, bilirubin 13 μ mol/l, protein 65 g/l, albumin 40 g/l, alkaline phosphatase 105 U/l, calcium 2.25 mmol/l, phosphate 0.8 mmol/l. Chest X-ray showed left lower lobe consolidation. Sputum microscopy showed gram positive cocci, no acid fast bacilli seen. Urinalysis negative.

A diagnosis of lobar pneumonia was made and he was started on ampicillin. In view of the possible dehydration an intravenous infusion was started and he was given Dextrose saline, 1 litre every four hours. Next day he was markedly improved, his fever was settling and he was less dyspnoeic. The following day, however, he complained of headache and nausea and later vomited his lunch. In the afternoon, he had become increasingly drowsy and confused.

On examination he was afebrile, pulse 100 per minute, blood pressure 140/85 mmHg, JVP not raised. There were crepitations at the left base. He had no neck stiffness, the pupils were equal and reacted to light and the fundi were normal. He had a generalized increase in muscle tone but no focal neurological signs could be demonstrated.

Investigations: Hb 14.0 g/dl, WBC 15 × 10^9/l, sodium 115 mmol/l, potassium 3.0 mmol/l, urea 2.5 m/l, PO_2 10.6 kPa (80 mmHg), PCO_2 5.6 kPa (42 mmHg). CSF was clear and contained 1 lymphocyte/mm^3.

1. What is the most likely diagnosis, and how would you confirm it?
2. How would you treat this?
3. What further investigations would you like to perform?

This man presents with a typical lobar pneumonia that responds well to antibiotics. His mental deterioration is associated with no focal neurological signs and no evidence of meningism. He is well oxygenated and the striking abnormality is his hyponatraemia. With his clinical state and fluid management he is unlikely to be sodium depleted and so water intoxication is probable. He has been given a considerable quantity of intravenous fluid since admission, but his renal function is good and his electrolyte imbalance is unlikely to be due to this alone. It is likely, then, that he is suffering from the syndrome of **inappropriate secretion of antidiuretic hormone**. To confirm this, plasma and urine osmolalities should be determined. The plasma osmolality will be low, but the kidney will not be producing an appropriately dilute urine so its osmolality will be higher than expected.

Treatment consists of **correcting the underlying cause**, and **fluid restriction**, a daily input of, say, 500 ml, to allow the body to lose its excess water. Giving saline usually results in its being rapidly excreted in the urine, but plasma sodium may be raised by causing a diuresis with frusemide and infusing 2N saline. These should be used with caution.

Although inappropriate ADH secretion can occur as a response to a chest infection, it is much more common a manifestation of an oat-cell bronchogenic carcinoma. This man must be further investigated with **sputum cytology** and, if necessary, following his recovery, by **bronchoscopy**.

If long-term treatment for inappropriate ADH secretion is necessary, fluid restriction is unpleasant for the patient and demeclocycline or lithium have been used which appear to decrease the renal response to ADH.

Case 57

A 33-year-old Russian engineer, who spent several months each year laying pipelines in Ethiopia, developed a flu-like illness one week after returning to the United Kingdom. This was of abrupt onset and consisted of malaise, headaches, myalgia, vomiting and upper abdominal discomfort. Physical examination revealed a fever of 39.5°C, slight icterus and some tenderness in the right hypochondrium. Urinalysis showed + + protein, + blood and the presence of bile.

Investigations showed: Hb 13.0 g/dl, WBC 6.0 × 10⁹/l, ESR 90 mm/h, aspartate transaminase 154 U/l, MSU showed 15–20 red blood cells per high powered field, but was otherwise normal. Stool and blood cultures negative, Brucella agglutinins, Widal and Paul–Bunnell tests all negative. The WR was positive and the chest X-ray normal.

No diagnosis was made and after four days he was treated empirically with ampicillin. His symptoms soon subsided but one week later he relapsed with identical complaints. His liver edge was just palpable, but physical examination was otherwise unchanged.

1. Give three likely diagnoses for this man's illness.
2. Suggest five further investigations.

This man, recently returned from East Africa, has a relapsing febrile illness, with evidence of hepatic and renal involvement. **Malaria** must be considered a strong possibility as the episodes of fever in this disease are not always regular, especially with falciparum malaria or a mixed infection. **Leptospirosis** can cause a similar picture; although patients usually get a leucocytosis, the white count is often initially low. Penicillin only affects the course of this disease if given very early. **Relapsing fever** (either tick- or louse-borne) might well present this way and penicillin does not prevent the relapses. Like the above diagnoses, it often has an abrupt onset. **Yellow fever** is less likely; it could easily have caused his initial illness and there may be an episode when fever remits, although this seldom lasts as long as a week. Other viral infections (hepatitis, dengue or haemorrhagic fevers) would be unlikely in view of the relapsing nature of the disease, and they are usually insidious in onset. Schistosomiasis is also an unlikely possibility, although there may be an episode of fever (with *S. mansoni* and not *S. haematobium*) some weeks after infection. Non-infective causes are also possible such as polyarteritis nodosa or a renal cell carcinoma with liver involvement.

Further investigations include the examination of **thick** and **thin blood films** for malarial parasites and *Borrelia* spirochaetes. In addition, *Leptospira* spirochaetes may be seen, but they are difficult to recognize. *Leptospira* is usually grown from the blood early in the illness (and his negative culture makes the diagnosis less likely). Later in the illness the organism may be grown from urine and repeat **urine culture** is necessary. Blood must also be sent for detection of **leptospira antibodies** by agglutination or complement fixation tests. **Yellow fever antibodies** must also be sought, but as they remain in high titre after an infection, it is necessary to demonstrate a rising titre. Blood should also be sent for HBsAg determination. *S. mansoni* would be diagnosed by finding **ova** in **stools or rectal biopsy**; serological methods are poor. Finally, if no cause has been found for this man's haematuria, an IVP and cystoscopy should be performed.

False positive WRs are common with any spirochaetal disease or with infections such as malaria or glandular fever. It may occur with autoimmune disease or occasionally after vaccination or any febrile illness. More specific tests such as **fluorescent Treponemal antibody test** and *Treponema pallidum* **immobilization tests** should be performed.

Case 58

A 48-year-old businessman went to see his doctor soon after returning home from a month's holiday in Sicily with his family. He did not feel any better for the break and had recently complained of vague headaches. Although he took little exercise and smoked and drank to excess he had never been seriously ill. He had recently lost a little weight.

On examination he was tanned. His blood pressure was 170/115 mmHg and, apart from a grade II hypertensive retinopathy, there were no other abnormal signs. The blood biochemistry showed urea 7.1 mmol/l, plasma sodium 147 mmol/l, potassium 2.7 mmol/l, bicarbonate 30 mmol/l, pH 7.5.

1. What is the most likely diagnosis?
2. What are two other possible diagnoses?
3. Suggests two tests that would confirm or refute your most likely diagnosis.

Aldosterone enhances sodium and potassium exchange in the distal convoluted tubule thereby causing hypokalaemia, alkalosis and a high urinary potassium excretion. The biochemical picture in this patient could, therefore, be explained by an inappropriate secretion of aldosterone (Conn's syndrome), secondary hyperaldosteronism (less likely in view of the high plasma sodium), or other steroids which have a mineralocorticoid action (Cushing's syndrome). In this patient, especially as he is a heavy smoker, an **ACTH secreting carcinoma of the bronchus** must be considered. His suntan might not be due solely to his recent holiday as hyperpigmentation is frequently found in extra-adrenal tumours. A chest X-ray must be performed and the diagnosis would be confirmed biochemically by finding raised **plasma cortisols** which would not be suppressed by a **dexamethasone suppression test**. Sputum cytology and possibly bronchoscopy may be indicated.

Conn's syndrome, in which plasma **aldosterone** levels are raised, with suppression of **plasma renin activity**, or **Cushing's syndrome** due to adrenal adenoma, adrenal hyperplasia or a pituitary basophil adenoma are less likely statistically, but nevertheless a skull X-ray and **CT brain scan** for evidence of pituitary enlargement is required. Occasionally accelerated hypertension may be accompanied by secondary hyperaldosteronism but in this case one would expect to find a more florid retinopathy. High plasma renin levels may occur in the absence of oedema and control of the hypertension results in disappearance of the secondary hyperaldosteronism. A hypokalaemic alkalosis is also seen with diarrhoea, excessive vomiting and diuretic or carbenoxolone therapy.

In Conn's syndrome the distinction between an adenoma and bilateral hyperplasia may be difficult. Patients with an adenoma tend to have a more severe biochemical disturbance with lower levels of plasma potassium, higher secretion rates of aldosterone and greater suppression of plasma renin activity. An adenoma may be localized by arteriography and/or adrenal venography. The latter may be a difficult procedure and carries the danger of adrenal infarction. Radioisotopic labelling of the tumour with ^{131}1-19-iodocholesterol (or alternative isotopes) may be attempted. In some cases computerized axial tomography and **adrenal MRI scanning** will identify a tumour. The definitive management of choice is removal of the tumour at laparotomy. Otherwise the hypertension may be controlled by spironolactone in conjunction with other antihypertensive drugs.

Case 59

A 37-year-old taxi driver was referred because of increasing difficulty in performing his job. He had been in good health all his life and had worked in the present job for nine years. Over the past six weeks, however, he had experienced increasing difficulty finding addresses even in areas he knew well. Despite resorting to a street map he was still often unable to get his bearings and following a number of complaints, he was now in danger of losing his job. His wife said the difficulty had started quite suddenly, but he had attributed this to fatigue and family worries; she was worried that he seemed relatively unconcerned. The symptoms appeared to vary from day to day, but the disability was greater at the time of referral than when the symptoms first appeared. He drank three pints of beer and smoked 15 cigarettes daily.

On examination he looked well. He was right-handed. Blood pressure was 130/84 mmHg; pulse 86 beats per minute and regular. There was no abnormality of the cardiovascular system, chest or abdomen. In the central nervous system he was alert and his memory, general knowledge and speech were normal, but some of his replies were not really appropriate. Examination of the cranial nerves was normal but neurophthalmic testing showed that whilst his visual fields were full and optic discs normal he could not generate an optic kinetic response to his right side. There was no abnormality of power, sensation, tone or reflexes. Both plantar responses were flexor. The following were normal or negative: blood count, ESR, urea and electrolytes, random blood sugar, serum calcium, liver enzymes, thyroid function tests, VDRL and TPHA. X-rays of the chest and skull were normal.

1. What is the localization of the lesion?
2. What is the likely cause?
3. Give two further investigations.
4. What visual field defect might you expect to find?

This man has a progressive functional disability involving the performance of a single acquired skill and affecting awareness of spatial relationships. This implies a lesion of the **non-dominant parietal lobe**, in his case probably the right side (since he is right-handed). Parietal lobe symptoms may vary from day to day but in this man the history is essentially progressive. An **intracranial tumour** is by far the most likely diagnosis. Unfortunately, 45% of all brain tumours in this age group are astrocytomas and a further 15% are metastases. A subdural haematoma would be considered in an older age group, even if there is no history of head injury, and meningiomas in females.

The non-dominant parietal lobe is necessary for appreciation of body image and orientation in extrapersonal space. When this is involved in a disease process, there may be difficulty in getting around, even in familiar surroundings, and inability to recognize landmarks or faces. With further damage, the patient may neglect his contralateral limbs, forgetting where they are, have difficulty in dressing or allow his limbs to lie in a bizarre position. Even though power may be preserved the affected limb may be ignored. These signs may be accompanied by a left inferior quadrant homonymous hemianopia and abnormal optic kinetic responses (the ability to generate a nystagmus to moving stripes on a drum or tape) are typical of parietal lobe tumours.

The relevant investigations in this patient are: An **EEG** which may show non-specific laterlizing abnormalities and **computerized axial tomographic brain scan** with enhancement will show a single lesion suggesting a tumour. If available, **MRI scan** of the brain will provide useful information. The shape of the lesion and the pattern of enhancement may indicate the likely pathology. Occasionally, multiple lesions are shown which would tend to support a diagnosis of metastases or granulomatous disease.

Case 60

A 47-year-old man was referred to medical outpatients by his GP. The GP felt that the man was depressed following the collapse six months previously of the family's painting and decorating business which the patient ran for several years with his father. He was now helping out at his brother's scrap yard.

The main complaint was of lethargy and frontal headaches occurring almost daily. He had lost interest in seeing friends and in sexual intercourse with his wife, and was waking early each morning with a feeling of anxiety. He was not eating well and only opening his bowels once each week. He had also started to limp on his left leg. He had no previous past medical history, took no medications and smoked 15 cigarettes daily. He drank 15 pints of beer each week.

On examination he looked depressed. He was pale but had no jaundice or lymphadenopathy. His teeth were in very poor condition. He had marked weakness of dorsiflexion of his left foot. The examination was otherwise unremarkable.

Investigations: Hb 9.8 g/dl, MCV 102 fl, platelets 342 × 10⁹/l, WBC 5.6 × 10⁹/l with normal differential, ESR 32 mm/l. Urea and electrolytes, liver function tests, thyroid function tests, calcium and phosphate and random glucose all normal. ECG and chest X-ray unremarkable. A contrast-enhanced computerized tomograph (CT scan) of the brain was normal.

1. What is the diagnosis?
2. Suggest three further tests which would help in making the diagnosis.
3. Suggest three important features in his management.

This case illustrates two important features. Firstly, an adequate occupational history is vital and secondly, although this patient is depressed, one should not rule out significant organic disease.

The patient presents with headaches, depression, anorexia, constipation and limping on his left leg. He has weakness of dorsiflexion of his left foot, probably due to a motor neuropathy and he is anaemic. An enhanced CT brain scan is normal making a **brain tumour** unlikely. He has worked in two professions which make his diagnosis of **chronic lead poisoning** more likely. Although modern paints are now lead-free, this was not always the case, and most lead poisoning in the UK now occurs in scrap metal or smelting workers. Domestic chronic lead-poisoning occurs in children, especially those living in old houses with lead water pipes. Acute lead poisoning can occur following accidental ingestion of fluid from car batteries.

Confirmatory investigations include **blood film** which will show **basophilic stippling of erythrocytes** and, because of interference with haem synthesis by lead, elevated urinary excretion of **5-amino-laevulinate** (ALA), an early and sensitive test. Urinary **coproporphyrin** is also increased. **Blood lead** concentration can be measured; in the UK, lead poisoning is a notifiable disease and work with lead is covered by strict regulations. Blood lead concentration should be below 4 mmol/l (800 μg/l) and levels above this are toxic.

This man's further management should include **avoidance of further lead exposure, notification of his condition** and treatment with **lead-chelating agents** such as dimercaprol, sodium calcium edetate (calcium EDTA) and penicillamine. If there is evidence of cerebral oedema, cotricosteroids and mannitol are often given, particularly in children.

Case 61

A 28-year-old woman journalist went to see her GP as she had been feeling unwell for six weeks with anorexia, lethargy, joint pains and a loss in weight of more than a stone.

On examination she was thin, pale, apyrexial and jaundiced. Her abnormal physical signs were confined to her abdomen, where she had a palpable liver 3 cm below her right costal margin, and the tip of the spleen was also palpable.

Investigations: Hb 11.0 g/dl, WBC 6 × 10⁹/l, bilirubin 34μ mol/l, alkaline phosphatase 140 U/l, aspartate transaminase 800 U/l, albumin 24 g/l, globulin 53 g/l.

1. What four further points from her history should be documented?
2. What is the most likely diagnosis?
3. What three further investigations would help you establish a diagnosis?

This young woman has liver disease and her biochemistry suggests hepatocellular damage rather than an obstructive pattern. It is very important to know whether she is a **heavy drinker** and also to obtain a **drug history** for possible toxic compounds. In addition, enquiry should be made about any episodes of **previous jaundice**.

Her clinical picture would fit with a **viral hepatitis**; probably type B in view of the length of symptoms and her arthritis (caused by immune complexes). A history of **contact or recent injections** should be sought.

Her raised globulin, however, suggests that the most likely diagnosis is **chronic active hepatitis**. There are several causes of this histological picture and it can occur after hepatitis caused by both type B and non A-non B viruses (now known to include hepatitis C, D, E and F). In addition, it can be precipitated by drugs or alcohol and rarer causes are Wilson's disease and alpha$_1$-antitrypsin deficiency. A large proportion of cases are of unknown aetiology (but perhaps autoimmune) and these 'lupoid' cases often present in young women.

Necessary investigations include a test for **hepatitis B surface antigen** which is positive in both the acute infection and those that progress to chronic hepatitis. Serum **protein electrophoresis** is necessary to define the cause of her hyperglobulinaemia and differential immunoglobulin levels may show the increased IgG that occurs in chronic active hepatitis. **Serum autoantibodies** should be looked for as in 'lupoid' chronic active hepatitis, anti-smooth muscle antibodies are found in 60% of cases and anti-mitochondrial antibodies in 25%. In addition, anti-nuclear antibody, Wasserman and rheumatoid factors may all be positive. If there is no obvious cause for her liver disease, or if she remains persistently HBsAg positive, then a **liver biopsy** should be performed after checking her **clotting studies**. Histologically the hallmark of chronic, active hepatitis is piecemeal necrosis. Chronic active hepatitis of any severity, especially if HBsAg negative, should be treated with steroids, whereas the benign **chronic persistent hepatitis** (which can give a similar clinical picture) needs no treatment. The value of steroids in HBsAg positive cases is debatable. Antiviral agents such as interferon are under trial.

Infectious mononucleosis can cause a hepatitis picture, but here the absence of pharyngitis and lymphadenopathy makes it unlikely. Primary biliary cirrhosis is unlikely to cause her biochemistry and she has no itching.

Case 62

A 75-year-old widow presented with a history of deteriorating vision in both eyes for the last three months and because of this she found it difficult to look after herself. She was on no medication and said she was otherwise well, but she recently had several falls resulting in a fracture of the neck of the right femur 18 months previously. This had been repaired surgically and following this she had problems with bedsores. Her falls were not associated with loss of consciousness, fits or vertigo. She had recovered without complication from pulmonary tuberculosis aged 21 years and she smoked 15–20 cigarettes a day.

On examination she was thin and frail and slightly paranoid. She saw 6/60 in each eye. She was unable to read any of the Ishihara colour test plates. The ocular media were clear and the optic discs normal. Visual fields showed bilateral central scotomas to red targets. Ocular examination was otherwise normal. Neurologically, muscle power in her limbs was quite good and tone was normal. She had absent ankle jerks, flexor plantar responses, other reflexes were normal. Joint position sensation was reduced in her feet and vibration could not be appreciated below her knees. Sensation in her arms was normal. Romberg's sign was mildly positive and she had some heel–shin ataxia.

Investigations: Hb 12.1 g/dl, WBC 7.9 × 10⁹/l, ESR 34 mm/h, PCV 41%, MCHC 19 g/dl, MCV 90 fl, urea and electrolytes normal.

1. Suggest two differential diagnoses.
2. What other information do you require?
3. What four investigations are necessary?

This patient had mild posterior column sensory loss and gross bilateral visual failure. The combination of bilateral poor acuity, colour loss and central scotomas suggest that this is due to optic nerve disease, in spite of the normal appearance of the optic discs. These signs suggest a **nutritional or toxic amblyopia** as the cause of her problems. Some elderly patients are often vague or fanciful about their diet and it requires persistence to get an **adequate dietary history** and details of their tobacco and alcohol consumption and medication. **B12 deficiency** is unlikely in view of the blood film, but **serum levels of B12** and **folate** must be measured. Some evidence of poor nutrition might be found in low levels of plasma proteins and the association of pernicious anaemia and gastric carcinomas must be remembered.

Nutritional amblyopia is not uncommon among elderly patients who do not look after themselves and it seems to be due to a combination of factors rather than purely to smoking or pernicious anaemia. The optic discs characteristically look normal. Visual recovery is usually dramatic over a period of weeks on vitamin supplements, B12 and a good diet.

Although the sensory signs would not support a compressive lesion affecting the optic nerves or chiasm as the cause of her visual failure, this must be considered and excluded by **skull X-rays** and a **CT scan**. The progressive nature of her symptoms suggests that optic nerve ischaemia is unlikely but occasionally a **carcinomatous optic neuropathy** can present like this and if this is considered, CSF must be obtained for cytology and a primary tumour (usually breast or lung) searched for in the normal way. In any patient with a combination of optic nerve disease and posterior column signs, **syphilis** must be excluded. With modern **serology** (FTA and TPHA) it is most unusual to get a negative blood serology and positive serology in the CSF, but this can occur rarely.

Case 63

A 34-year-old West Indian was admitted to hospital with a complaint of progressive breathlessness over the previous four months. He also had an unproductive cough. He complained that since arriving in England three years before, his hands had become very painful and pale in cold weather.

On examination the abnormal findings were confined to the hands and the chest. In the chest, areas of bronchial breathing and aegophony were noted over the mid zones, with fine crepitations at both bases.

Investigations: Hb, WBC and ESR normal. Chest X-ray showed patchy shadowing in both mid zones and bases, FEV$_1$ 1200 ml, FVC 1400 ml, arterial blood gases—PaO_2 8.6 kPa (65 mmHg), $PaCO_2$ 5.3 kPa (40 mmHg), pH 7.4.

1. What is the most likely diagnosis?
2. What three abnormal findings may have been discovered on examination of the hands?
3. What three further investigations would you perform?

The history of cold intolerance in this patient is strongly suggestive of Raynaud's phenomenon. The primary or idiopathic form of the disease may occur in isolation; however, Raynaud's phenomenon may be associated with several conditions including thromboangitis obliterans, trauma, cervical rib, the collagen diseases, cold agglutinins and cryoglobulinaemia.

The progressive history of breathlessness, together with evidence of a restrictive defect in pulmonary function, associated with hypoxia without hypercapnia, suggests a diffusion abnormality for which there are many possible causes such as fibrosing alveolitis, sarcoid, scleroderma, multiple pulmonary emboli, and so on.

The co-existence of pulmonary disease and Raynaud's phenomenon strongly suggests **scleroderma** and, in addition to the signs of Raynaud's phenomenon in the hands, **skin thickening** with **tethering of the skin, subcutaneous calcification** and **telangiectasia** should be looked for and a history of **dysphagia** sought.

Further investigations might include measurement of **transfer factor** (diffusion capacity for carbon monoxide) which would be decreased, a **barium swallow** for evidence of oesophageal involvement, and a **skin biopsy** for histological evidence of scleroderma. **Antinuclear antibodies** are present in 70%; **anti-Scl-70 antibodies** are present in 20%. The **CREST** syndrome (**C**alcinosis, **R**aynaud's phenomenon, o**E**sophageal involvement, **S**clerodactyly and **T**elangiectasia) is associated with anti-centromere antinuclear antibodies in the blood.

No treatment has been shown to influence the progress of scleroderma; mean five-year survival is 50%.

Case 64

A 24-year-old army private was brought to casualty because of severe headache, nausea and vomiting. These symptoms had developed five days previously during a three-week field training exercise and had become progressively more severe. Fellow soldiers who had been sharing the same tents were well. He smoked 20 cigarettes a day and usually drank 10 pints of beer a week, but had taken no alcohol for three weeks. He used a salbutamol inhaler intermittently for mild exercise-induced asthma and had no relevant past medical history. He denied ever having used intravenous drugs.

On examination he looked unwell and had a fever of 38°C. He had marked photophobia and meningism, as evidenced by a rigid neck and positive Kernig's sign. Fundoscopy and the rest of the neurological examination were normal. He had several tattoos. There was marked bruising affecting both legs, thighs and forearms. His conjunctivae were injected and he looked mildly jaundiced. The remainder of the examination was unremarkable.

Investigations: Hb 15.6 g/dl, WBC 17 × 10⁹/1, platelets 67 × 10⁹/1, ESR 87 mm/h, prothrombin time 28 s (control 15 s), activated partial thromboplastin time 67 s (control 35 s). Urea 18.9 mmol/l, creatinine 160 μmol/l, sodium 130 mmol/l, potassium 5.2 mmol/l, glucose 5.1 mmol/l, bilirubin 57 μmol/l, aspartate amino transferase (AST) 86 IU/l (normal < 35), alkaline phosphatase 421 IU/l (normal < 300), albumin 42 g/dl. Monospot test negative. ECG and chest X-ray normal. Urine dipstick revealed 2 + proteinuria, 2 + blood. Examination of the cerebrospinal fluid: opening pressure 19 cm CSF, clear and colourless, RBC 4/mm³, WBC 18 lymphocytes/mm³, protein 0.44 g/dl, glucose 3.6 mmol/l.

1. What is the most likely diagnosis?
2. Suggest three further investigations to make the diagnosis.
3. What is the treatment and are there any complications of this?
3. Suggest two alternative diagnoses.

This young man presents with hepatitis, a lymphocytic meningitis and renal impairment. He has thrombocytopenia and clotting derangements suggestive of disseminated intravascular coagulation. The most likely diagnosis is **leptospirosis (Weil's disease)** caused by infection with *Leptospira icterohaemorrhagicae*, present in water contaminated by rodent urine. Soldiers are the group most commonly affected by this disease in the UK; other groups at risk are farmers, sewage workers, abattoir workers and veterinarians. The disease occurs in two phases. Following an incubation period of 10 days, there is a 'leptospiraemic phase' which lasts one week, followed by an 'immune phase' during which 50% suffer meningism; one-third of those with meningism have a lymphocytic meningitis and raised CSF protein. There may be an asymptomatic period of several days between the phases. Bleeding complications and myocarditis are not uncommon. The diagnosis is made clinically and supported serologically, by complement fixation and by culture of the spirochaete.

Anti-Leptospira IgM can be detected, and a **complement fixation test** and **Schuffner agglutination test** can be carried out. In the first week, **blood** and **CSF culture** may be positive; in weeks 2–5, **urine culture** is more often positive. Treatment is **supportive** (e.g. dialysis for renal failure) and **benzylpenicillin** is given, or erythromycin in penicillin-sensitive individuals. Tetracycline and chloramphenicol can be used. The **Jarisch–Herxheimer reaction** of occasionally fatal cardiovascular collapse is a rare complication of therapy, occuring possibly as a result of massive release of endotoxin. Most patients recover fully from leptospirosis.

Other infectious diseases may cause this presentation. **Lyme disease** caused by another spirochaete, *Borrelia burgdoferi* can produce a similar illness. This follows a bite by the tick Ixodes, usually in forested areas. It has 3 stages: 50% have erythema migrans, 2–30 days after the tick bite, with fever and non-specific constitutional symptoms; 1–4 months later come cardiac and central nervous system complications (e.g. myocarditis, heart block and lymphocytic meningitis); finally, 10% develop chronic erosive arthritis. Diagnosis is serological and treatment is with tetracycline and a penicillin. **Viral hepatitis (A or B), E-B virus, CMV, toxoplasma** and **human immunodeficiency virus (HIV)** may produce this picture although the Monospot test is negative. These can be diagnosed serologically. HepBsAg and Hep A IgM should be checked.

Case 65

A 24-year-old newspaper reporter came to casualty with a three week history of recurrent sore throat, nocturnal sweats, dry cough, occipital headaches and aching muscles. His headaches were on two occasions preceded by episodes of blurred vision. Three days before admission he developed difficulty in passing urine which progressed to urinary retention. At this time he also developed paraesthesiae, weakness in his feet and legs and unsteadiness of gait.

The previous year he had been admitted to hospital with concussion from a car crash. His father had been treated for pulmonary tuberculosis eight years previously.

He was admitted to hospital and catheterized. Over the next two days the paraesthesiae rose to involve the trunk and lower chest and his weakness and unsteadiness progressed so that he could not walk.

On examination, he was pyrexial (37.5°C) with a furred tongue, large tonsils and enlarged lymph glands in his neck. The rest of the abnormal findings were confined to the nervous system. Cranial nerves were normal. Despite weakness in both legs, he had normal tone in all four limbs and co-ordination of the arms was normal. His leg tendon reflexes were increased with extensor plantar reflexes; abdominal reflexes were diminished and cremasteric reflexes were absent. All modalities of sensation were impaired up to T5.

1. Give four possible diagnoses.
2. Give five important investigations.

This young man has a transverse myelitis. However, he has had symptoms above T5 (his two episodes of blurred vision) which suggests a more generalized disease, quite possibly infection in view of the prodromal illness. It is essential with his family history to rule out **tuberculous meningitis** and a **tuberculous abscess** compressing the spinal cord at T5. A malignant **space-occupying lesion** must be considered even in the absence of root pain and spinal tenderness. The clinical picture is extremely acute for **disseminated sclerosis,** which in its acute form may be associated with optic neuritis (Devic's syndrome). **Syphilis** may cause a similar picture, but there is no history of contact and no evidence of the rash associated with secondary syphilis. **Exanthemata** can cause a transverse myelitis, and in this context with lymphadenopathy and large exudative tonsils, infectious mononucleosis is a strong possibility and carries a good prognosis. Measles and mumps are also rare causes and a transverse myelitis is sometimes seen following vaccination. Infection with **human immunodeficiency virus** (**HIV**) can produce transverse myelitis, either during acute seroconversion or during the chronic phase.

Examination of the CSF is mandatory in this case for acid fast bacilli, culture, examination of cells, protein and glucose. A **chest X-ray** may show pulmonary tuberculosis and an **X-ray of the dorsal spine** may reveal a tuberculous abscess or bone destruction by a space-occupying lesion. **Syphilis serology** should be carried out in all patients suffering from neurological disease and in this case, a **Paul–Bunnell** and **titre for EB virus** should be performed. If cord compression is suspected, a **myelogram** should be performed and the contrast medium introduced when the lumbar puncture is performed. **MRI scanning** is an excellent technique for imaging the spinal cord.

If other tests are negative and after appropriate counselling an **anti-HIV antibody test** should be considered.

Case 66

A 25-year-old airline steward was sent to his GP with low back pain, worse in the mornings, and pain in his left knee. This had started three weeks previously and more recently the backache had radiated to his right leg, and he had developed sore eyes. On direct questioning, he admitted to an episode of diarrhoea about four weeks before. Both his grandfather and uncle had suffered from back trouble.

On examination he had limitation of movement of the lower back due to pain and his left knee was swollen and tender. There was bilateral iritis. Physical examination was otherwise normal.

X-ray of this man's sacroiliac joints showed sclerosis and erosion of the lower joint margins. X-ray of his lumbar spine was normal.

1. What is the most likely diagnosis?
2. Name four other possible diagnoses.
3. Name three non-musculoskeletal complications of your initial diagnosis.

This man has the features of **ankylosing spondylitis**. As well as the typical backache and sacroiliitis, this disease may have a peripheral arthritis (usually of the larger joints), iritis, plantar fasciitis and Achilles tendinitis. It has a familial tendency.

Other causes of a seronegative arthritis must, however, be considered—they can all cause back pain and iritis. His episode of diarrhoea raises the possibility of **Reiter's disease** which may occur after *Shigella*, *Salmonella* and *Yersinia* infections, as well as following non-specific urethritis. In this condition, however, sacro-iliitis is a feature of severe disease and generally occurs late. Gastrointestinal infections can also cause a reactive arthritis without the other features of Reiter's disease. This man's diarrhoea could also be a sign of early **ulcerative colitis** or **Crohn's disease**, both of which may be accompanied by a flitting monoarthritis of large joints or by a picture identical to ankylosing spondylitis. The arthropathy may precede the development of other symptoms, as it can also with **psoriatic arthropathy**. This can take several forms, often being an asymmetrical polyarthritis, an arthritis of distal interphalangeal joints, a picture identical to rheumatoid arthritis or, less commonly, a mutilating arthritis. On occasion, however, it can mimic ankylosing spondylitis. A rare cause of sacroiliitis is Whipple's disease. Behçet's disease is excluded by the absence of buccal or genital ulceration and other features of the disease, and rheumatoid disease does not cause iritis (it causes a scleritis) and the joint distribution would be most unusual.

Most causes of sacroiliitis are associated with an increased incidence of the major histocompatibility antigen HLA-B27. This occurs in 8% of Caucasian controls and its incidence varies from 90% in ankylosing spondylitis to 40% in the central form of psoriatic arthritis. There is no correlation with rheumatoid disease or Behçet's syndrome.

Complications of ankylosing spondylitis include **aortic incompetence** and **cardiac conduction defects**. About 1% of sufferers develop a characteristic **upper zone pulmonary fibrosis**. Another rare complication is secondary **amyloid disease**.

Case 67

A 46-year-old housewife was sent to medical outpatients by her GP. She had a three month history of weight loss, having lost 10 kg despite a good appetite. She was constipated and had been having frequent frontal headaches. Her menstrual periods had become irregular. At the age of 25 she had undergone surgery for a bleeding duodenal ulcer, but still needed to take intermittent courses of ranitidine for recurrent episodes of severe dyspepsia occuring every few months. Her mother died at the age of 55 from renal failure.

On examination she was thin and anxious. She had a fine tremor of the outstretched hands and lid lag. There was no goitre. Pulse 110/min, regular, BP 115 / 70 mmHg. She had a well-healed vertical midline abdominal incision. Examination was otherwise unremarkable.

Investigations: full blood count and film, urea and electrolytes and fasting glucose and lipids normal. ESR 23 mm/hour. Albumin 42 g/l, corrected total calcium 3.4 mmol/l, phosphate 0.3 mmol/l (confirmed on an uncuffed sample). Free thyroxine 40 pmol/l, TSH < 0.05 IU/l. Chest and abdominal X-rays, ECG and urine normal. Pregnancy test negative. Abdominal ultrasound normal.

1. What is the unifying diagnosis?
2. Suggest four important further investigations.
3. Is there a genetic basis for this disease?

This woman presents with a history of weight loss despite a good appetite. Few conditions produce this combination and include thyrotoxicosis, untreated diabetes mellitus and some early lymphoproliferative disorders and leukaemias. Clinical examination and thyroid function tests confirm thyrotoxicosis, while blood glucose, full blood count and film are normal. In addition she has constipation and frontal headaches, with marked hypercalcaemia and hypophosphataemia. Although thyrotoxicosis can cause hypercalcaemia, it is rarely of this degree and other causes such as hyperparathyroidism should be considered. There is a family history of renal failure, possibly related to hypercalcaemia. There is also a history of recurrent severe dyspepsia despite previous peptic ulcer surgery: this suggests either failed surgery, or a condition of recurrent peptic ulceration, such as Zollinger–Ellison syndrome, caused by a slow-growing malignancy of gastrin-secreting pancreatic G cells. The unifying diagnosis in this case is **multiple endocrine neoplasia syndrome type I** (**MEN**-I); this would explain simultaneous disease affecting thyroid, parathyroid and pancreatic glands.

Further investigations should be aimed at all endocrine organs which could be involved, which are in order of frequency: parathyroid 95%, pituitary 70%, pancreas 50%, adrenal 40%, thyroid 20%. Adenomas may be single or multiple, functional or non-functional, or the glands may be hyperplastic. Investigations should thus include **parathormone** level (if detectable at this degree of hypercalcaemia, this supports autonomous secretion), and **pituitary function tests**, both baseline (Prolactin, ACTH, LH, FSH, etc.) and dynamic. **Gastrin** levels should be checked, and a **CT scan** or if available, **magnetic resonance imaging** (MRI) of affected glands will help to identify adenomas. Radioisotope scanning and selective venous catheterization and sampling is occasionally necessary. Treatment of adenomas is surgical, while thyrotoxicosis if due to hyperplasia may be treated medically with radioiodine ablation although this is more appropirate in an older patient, or carbimazole and thyroxine replacement ('block and replace').

MEN-I is inherited as an **autosomal dominant** condition. The affected gene has been localized to the long arm of chromosome 11, located close to oncogenes coding for proteins with fibroblastic growth activity. Relatives should be screened biochemically (e.g. calcium estimation). Genetic markers for screening are being sought.

Case 68

A 50-year-old woman was sent to hospital by her employers, the nuns of a convent where she had lived and worked as a domestic servant since she was a girl of 15.

The patient was mentally subnormal, but was capable of looking after herself and doing simple work. She was cheerful and uncomplaining, but the mother superior said she had become more lethargic and easily tired for the previous three months. The patient suffered from grand mal epilepsy for which she took phenobarbitone and phenytoin, but had not taken these regularly and had not bothered to visit her doctor.

On examination she was very pale, and had the physical signs of Down's syndrome. She had bad teeth, hyperplastic gums, but no lymphadenopathy. She had crepitations at both lung bases and ankle oedema. In her abdomen her liver was not palpable, but the spleen could be tipped.

A blood examination showed: Hb 4.0 g/dl, WBC 3.0×10^9/l, 50% lymphocytes, 38% polymorphs, 6% monocytes and 6% eosinophils. Platelets 40×10^9/l, MCV 108 fl, MCHC 20 g/dl.

1. What are the two most likely diagnoses?
2. Suggest two other possible diagnoses.
3. Suggest the three most helpful investigations.

The two most likely diagnoses in this patient are **folate deficiency** due to poor dietary intake and anticonvulsant therapy, or **pernicious anaemia**. Mild degrees of splenomegaly can be associated with any cause of severe megaloblastic anaemia. Another possible, but rare, diagnosis is an aleukaemic presentation of **acute myeloid** or **lymphatic leukaemia**, and patients with Down's syndrome do have an increased incidence of acute myeloid and lymphatic leukaemia. The anaemia of myxoedema is normally normochromic and normocytic, but 15% of patients have an associated B12 deficiency due to pernicious anaemia. Down's syndrome sufferers are more prone to hypothyroidism. Tuberculosis can cause macrocytosis, but such a severe anaemia in both these causes would not occur without a co-existing deficiency state. Myelofibrosis would not normally fit into this clinical picture, particularly with such a relatively small spleen.

The three most helpful investigations would be **a bone marrow, red cell folate**, and **serum B12**. Further investigations might include a Schilling test and thyroid function.

The patient had, in fact, pernicious anaemia.

Case 69

A woman of 55 attended the chest clinic. 30 years before she had had a thoracoplasty for pulmonary tuberculosis. She smoked heavily and always had a productive cough. Apart from several haemoptyses over the years she had been well, but recently her shortness of breath had become worse and she had had a further haemoptysis. Her left wrist was swollen and tender and she was taking aspirin to relieve the pain.

On examination she was cyanosed, dyspnoeic and febrile. There was a right thoracoplasty scar and the trachea deviated to the right. In the right upper zone there was dullness to percussion, an area of bronchial breathing and coarse crepitations. Her fingers were clubbed.

1. Suggest two possible causes for her repeated haemoptyses over the years.
2. What are the four possible causes for her present illness?
3. Give two reasons for her swollen wrist.

By the removal of several ribs a thoracoplasty allowed the chest wall to collapse and obliterate a tuberculous cavity. It was an effective and time-honoured treatment that has now been superseded by modern chemotherapy but, nevertheless, there are still many people who have had their pulmonary tuberculosis treated this way. Residual **bronchiectasis** is common in these patients and this, or a reactivation of their quiescent **tuberculosis**, may lead to fresh haemoptyses. Rarely fungi colonize damaged parts of the lung and the resulting mycetoma will manifest itself by recurrent haemoptyses.

This woman now has a febrile illness associated with signs of collapse and consolidation in the right lung. An **acute infection** is the most likely diagnosis but **bronchial carcinoma**, **pulmonary embolus** or reactivation of the **tuberculosis** must be considered.

The wrist swelling might be due to a **tuberculous arthritis** or **hypertrophic pulmonary osteoarthropathy**. This is frequently associated with bronchial carcinoma but is sometimes also seen with long-standing bronchiectasis, or other conditions including Crohn's disease, primary biliary cirrhosis and cyanotic congenital heart disease.

Case 70

A 24-year-old student went to see his general practitioner with a three week history of low back pain, especially in the mornings. On questioning, he admitted that he had had difficulty playing games at school through back trouble, but until the present exacerbation this had improved. In addition, he had visited his general practitioner occasionally with abdominal discomfort and diarrhoea for which he had been given Colofac with no real success.

On examination, he was pyrexial and anaemic. The only other abnormal physical sign was that he had a tender palpable mass in the right iliac fossa. Rectal examination and sigmoidoscopy were normal. He had tenderness on flexion of his lumbosacral spine.

Initial investigations: Hb 9.0 g/dl, ESR 60 mm/h, WBC 10.0 × 10⁹/l, stool culture and microscopy negative.

1. Give your diagnosis and two other possibilities.
2. Suggest five further investigations.

The most likely situation in this young man is inflammatory disease of the bowel associated with inflammatory joint disease affecting his lumbosacral spine. This association points towards **Crohn's disease** which may present as a mass in the right iliac fossa. **Ileocaecal tuberculosis** may also present in this fashion if there is associated tubercular disease of the spine. The only malignant type of disease which is likely to present in this way and in this age group would be a **lymphoma of the small bowel** metastasizing to the lumbosacral spine. Ulcerative colitis may also present with inflammatory bowel disease and spondylitis. It is extremely rare, however, for it to present as a mass in the right iliac fossa and it is also very unusual to have a normal sigmoidoscopy. An appendix abscess could present in this way and also actinomycosis, but neither could explain the back symptoms.

Investigations must include a **chest X-ray, X-ray of the lumbosacral spine and sacroiliac joints** to look for spondylitis or possible tuberculous or lymphomatous involvement of these areas. **Barium studies** should be performed to look for disease in the bowel, in particular the ileocaecal area. A **rectal biopsy** might show typical features of Crohn's disease and if tuberculosis is really suggested, then acid fast bacilli should be sought with cultures of stool, early morning urine and gastric washings. **Colonoscopy** with **biopsies** may provide the answer. If these do not give a firm diagnosis, **laparotomy** may be necessary. An isotopic bone scan might be helpful in the further investigation of his back symptoms.

Case 71

A 57-year-old man was brought to casualty by two police officers who had found him collapsed on the pavement. He was known to have no fixed abode. No further information was available, and the patient could not give a history.

On examination he looked unkempt and smelt heavily of alcohol. He was conscious, self-ventilating and moving all limbs, but was drowsy and mumbling incoherently. He had no meningism and no abnormal focal neurological signs. Pulse 90/min, regular, BP 160/100 mmHg. Examination of the heart, lungs and abdomen was normal.

Investigations: Hb 14.3 g/dl, MCV 102 fl, WBC 10 × 10^9/l, platelets 274 × 10^9/l, urea 8mmol/l, sodium 145 mmol/l, potassium 5 mmol/l, glucose 5 mmol, plasma osmolality 393 mOsm/l, blood ethanol concentration 15 mmol/l. Chest X-ray and ECG normal.

The patient was diagnosed as having acute alcohol intoxication and admitted to the overnight observation ward. He was given a parenteral multivitamin preparation which included thiamine and oral chlormethiazole. The following morning he was alert and co-operative, and ate a good breakfast. He accepted the offer to see the social worker who was due to see him that evening. During that afternoon, he became once again progressively more unwell with confusion, headache and he became photophobic. He was noted to be hyperventilating and arterial blood gases on air showed: PaO$_2$ 11 kPa (83 mmHg), PaCO$_2$ 2.9 kPa (22 mmHg), pH 7.1. A CT brain scan was carried out which was normal, as was examination of cerebrospinal fluid. The following morning, he had become totally blind.

1. What is the diagnosis.
2. Why did his condition deteriorate?
3. Suggest three further vital investigations.
4. What is the treatment?
5. Suggest four further causes of impaired consciousness in such a patient.

The differential diagnosis of altered consciousness in a patient with known or suspected alcohol abuse is a very common and important clinical problem. The initial diagnosis of ethanol intoxication was supported by a high blood ethanol level. Subsequently, there was headache, photophobia, metabolic acidosis, with a normal CT brain scan and CSF, and finally blindness. The inital plasma osmolality was measured as 393 mOsm/l. It is possible to estimate the plasma osmolality as approximately:

[Plasma osmolality = 2 × (Na + K) + urea + glucose + ethanol]

(which in this case is 328 mOsm/l). There is thus a discrepancy between measured and estimated plasma osmolality of 65 mOsm/l. This suggests the presence of another osmotically-active agent at high concentration. Such agents include salicylate, ketone bodies, methanol and ethylene glycol. Further vital investigations therefore include a repeat **blood glucose**, **urinary ketones**, urgent **blood** and **urine drug screen**, and measurement of **bicarbonate** and **chloride** to establish the **anion gap**.

The diagnosis in this case was **methanol poisoning**. This is metabolized by hepatic alcohol dehydrogenase to methanal (formaldehyde) and methanoate (formate). In the presence of competing ethanol, this conversion is slow since the affinity for methanol of alcohol dehydrogenase is 15% that of ethanol. When ethanol levels have fallen, the reaction proceeds. These toxic metabolites cause headache, vomiting, photophobia and a marked metabolic acidosis. In cases of severe intoxication, respiratory failure and death may ensue. Visual disturbances are almost universal and range from blurred vision to total blindness due to direct retinal and optic nerve damage. Chronic methanol abuse is associated with papilloedema and optic atrophy. Treatment is with **intravenous ethanol** or **dialysis**. **Folinic acid** may prevent ocular toxicity.

In an alcoholic with impaired consciousness, one should always consider:

1. **Intracranial pathology**: meningitis, encephalitis, cerebrovascular accident, postictal state, subdural or extradural haematomas, space-occupying lesion such as abscess or tumour.
2. **Metabolic derangement**: hypoglycaemia, hepatic encephalopathy, Wernicke's encephalopathy, septicaemia, drug overdose, diabetic ketoacidosis.
3. **Direct alcohol effect**: acute intoxication, acute withdrawal.
4. **Hypothermia**.

Case 72

A woman of 68 (a well-known public figure) was referred for a medical opinion by the ophthalmic department who had noticed her to have abnormal pupils at a routine examination. The patient said her only complaint was some tingling and numbness in the right index and middle fingers for two or three years and she sometimes had difficulty in picking up small objects with that hand. A doctor had told her that her pupils were abnormal at least ten years previously. Almost 30 years ago she had had a partial thyroidectomy for a toxic goitre but had never had anything else wrong with her.

Abnormal findings were limited to the nervous system. Her pupils were small and showed no reaction to light, but reacted to accommodation. The other cranial nerves were normal. Her ankle jerks and left knee jerk were absent but all sensory modalities were normal in her legs. There was some generalized loss of sensation in the right thumb, index and middle fingers with slight wasting of the adductor pollicus brevis. Otherwise there were no abnormal findings.

1. Give the two most likely explanations for her pupil abnormalities.
2. What is the probable cause of the symptoms in her right hand, and give two useful investigations in your management.

This woman's pupillary reactions could be due to either **Argyll Robertson** pupils or bilateral **Adie's tonic** pupils. The former are found in tertiary syphilis and rarely in diabetes mellitus. Adie's pupils can be bilateral in a substantial number of patients and, although initially they are dilated, with time they become miosed. There is usually some preservation of the light reflex but this can be difficult to see and careful examination of the near reflex is necessary to pick up the tonic response. The lesion lies in the ciliary ganglion. Adie's pupils are frequently associated with loss of knee and ankle jerks and sometimes upper limb reflexes, but there is never any sensory disturbance. The diagnosis can be confirmed by demonstrating hypersensitivity to weak pilocarpine drops. The diagnosis of Adie's pupils in this patient spared her a lumbar puncture which would otherwise have been a necessity.

Her hand symptoms were due to a **carpal tunnel syndrome**. This was confirmed by showing delayed conduction on **electromyography**. A carpal tunnel syndrome can be associated with myxoedema and in view of her previous partial thyroidectomy, **thyroid function tests** were done which were, however, normal. A Horner's syndrome can follow thyroid surgery, but of course these pupils retain normal light and near reflexes.

Case 73

A 22-year-old girl was well until 12 months before, when she started to become short of breath on effort and latterly this had been associated with tightness across the upper chest. There was no history of rheumatic heart disease and she had never been cyanosed. Five years previously she had applied to work as a cook in a London hospital and no abnormality had been found at the medical examination. She did not smoke and drank only rarely. Her mother was alive and well, but her father had collapsed and died suddenly when she was a young girl. She had two younger brothers who were both well.

On examination, she was not anaemic or clubbed. The pulse was 80 per minute, regular with normal upstroke. The blood pressure was 120/70 mmHg, and her venous pressure was not raised. The cardiac apex was not displaced and was double in character. Cardiac auscultation revealed normal first and second heart sounds and both a fourth heart sound and late systolic murmur were audible at the apex. The lung fields were clear.

Investigations: Chest X-ray showed a normal heart size. ECG showed Q-waves in leads V2–V6 with changes of left ventricular hypertrophy and T-wave inversion. Full blood count, serum lipids, thyroid function and syphilis serology were normal.

1. What is the diagnosis?
2. How would you confirm this and what abnormalities would you expect to find?
3. What is the cause of her double apical impulse?
4. How would you treat the girl?

This girl presents with symptoms of angina pectoris at an unusually early age and no risk factors apart, perhaps, from her father's early death. This makes her angina unlikely to be due to coronary artery disease and the abnormalities on examination support this. She has signs typical of **hypertrophic obstructive cardiomyopathy (HOCM)**, a disorder which must always be considered in the differential diagnosis of angina.

A jerky pulse may occur due to a rapid initial upstroke followed by the development of left ventricular outflow obstruction causing a small sustained second component. The double apical impulse is a palpable atrial filling thrust—increased to overcome the resistance to left ventricular filling caused by the cardiomyopathy. The late systolic murmur is due to outflow tract obstruction distorting the mitral valve and causing regurgitation.

Diagnostic confirmation is usually via **echocardiography** which may reveal:

1. A greatly thickened septum (> 1.3 cm) with a ratio of septal to posterior wall thickness of > 1.5 (asymmetrical septal hypertrophy, ASH).
2. Systolic anterior motion of the anterior mitral valve leaflet (SAM).
3. Mid-systolic closure of the aortic valve.

It will rarely be necessary to proceed to left ventricular angiography which shows a bent slit-like, 'tear-drop' left ventricular cavity.

The mainstay of treatment of angina in HOCM is with **beta-adrenergic blocking drugs** which allow improved ventricular filling and decrease the outflow tract obstruction. Vasodilators such as nitrates should be avoided as these cause peripheral venous pooling. Many patients improve symptomatically on therapy, but there is no definite evidence that it prevents ventricular arrhythmias and sudden death to which they are prone. Some groups of patients with ventricular arrhythmias are treated with **amiodarone** and there is some evidence that this is associated with greater survival. HOCM is usually inherited as an autosomal dominant condition and this girl's father no doubt died suddenly because he was also a sufferer. The rest of the family should also be screened with echocardiography. The genetic abnormality in HOCM has been localized.

If patients do not respond to beta-adrenergic blockers and have persistent outflow tract gradients, then surgery can be performed to resect the septal hypertrophy. Mitral valve replacement may also be necessary. The operation has a significant mortality and morbidity.

Case 74

The patient, a 45-year-old salesman, had been admitted to hospital with an attack of left sided pleuritic pain, which had lasted for 24 hours and then subsided. At that time, he had been well apart from severe but fleeting pains in his wrists which he had attributed to 'rheumatism'. He smoked 10 cigarettes a day.

Examination at that time showed no abnormalities apart from the signs of a small left sided pleural effusion and mild synovial swelling in both wrists. There was no evidence of venous thrombosis in the legs.

Investigation at that time showed a normal blood count, electrolytes and sputum culture. Sputum cytology was negative for malignant cells. Aspiration of the pleural effusion demonstrated clear yellow fluid, protein content 35 g/l, which contained no cells and was sterile on culture (including Löwenstein–Jensen culture). X-ray of the wrists was normal and chest X-ray showed the small effusion, but was otherwise normal. He was followed up in the chest clinic and the radiological appearances remained unchanged.

Four months later, he was admitted as an emergency in a confused state. He had become increasingly agitated over three days and was expressing paranoid ideas about his wife's infidelity with the local greengrocer. The patient was afebrile with no papilloedema or neurological signs.

Subsequent investigation showed: Hb 13.4 g/dl, WBC 3.0 × 10⁹/l, platelets 320 × 10⁹/l, ESR 80 mm/h. Urea and electrolytes were normal. Blood sugar 6.4 mmol/l. Calcium 2.38 mmol/l, WR was negative. CT brain scan was normal. Lumbar puncture was performed and showed an opening pressure of 14 cm CSF. Examination showed 40 lymphocytes per cubic millimetre, no malignant cells, gram stain negative, protein 0.8 g/l, sugar 5 mmol/l. The chest X-ray appearances of the pleural effusion were unchanged. No parenchymal lung lesion was seen.

1. What is the diagnosis?
2. Give one investigation to confirm it.

WBC 3.0×10^9/l, platelets 320×10^9/l

The cause of this patient's pleural effusion remained unknown despite investigation. Pneumonia and pulmonary infarction are unlikely, but malignancy and tuberculosis are both very real possibilities, especially in view of the subsequent confusional state. Tuberculous effusions may be difficult to diagnose and positive culture may only be obtained in 25% of cases. However, the subsequent mental picture and CSF findings are unlikely to be explained by tuberculous meningitis, although cultures for tuberculosis should certainly be set up. A malignant effusion is unlikely in view of the static nature of the chest X-ray and negative sputum cytology.

There are a number of causes of mental changes in patients with carcinoma of the bronchus, including frontal lobe secondaries, hyponatraemia (usually due to inappropriate ADH secretion), hypercalcaemia (bone secondaries or ectopic parathyroid hormone production), or a non-metastatic encephalopathy. Painful wrists in a patient with a possible pulmonary neoplasm suggests hypertrophic pulmonary osteoarthropathy, but X-ray of the wrists did not show subperiosteal new bone formation. However, arthritis and pleural involvement raise the possibility of a connective tissue disorder, which taken in conjunction with a confusional state and a mild leucopenia, is strongly suggestive of **systemic lupus erythematosus**. This should be confirmed by the finding of raised titre of **anti-DNA antibodies**.

Cerebral involvement in systemic lupus erythematosus is common, usually manifesting as epilepsy or psychiatric changes. This latter occurs in up to 60% of patients and may vary from mild behavioural disturbances to a florid psychosis. The pathological change is thought to be a vasculitis of the cerebral arteries and normally responds well to steroids. Other neurological manifestations include peripheral neuropathy, myelopathy, hemiplegia and chorea.

Case 75

A 72-year-old retired school teacher had been on 10 mg prednisone daily for two years to control her temporal arteritis when she was seen complaining of sudden severe backache which had started two days previously. The pain was severe, radiating to her left groin and worse on coughing or movement.

Apart from her temporal arteritis she had always been well and took no drugs other than her steroids. She did not smoke or drink.

When examined she seemed well and cheerful. There was some pallor of her mucous membranes and tenderness over her spine in the area of T10 to T11. The spleen could just be tipped but otherwise examination was normal.

Investigations showed: chest X-ray normal; spinal X-rays showed collapse of the vertebral bodies of T10 and T11; Hb 9.9 g/dl, WBC 9.0 × 10⁹/l, ESR 8 mm/h, PCV 0.31, MCV 120 fl, MCHC 20 mmol/l, reticulocytes 7%, platelets 273 × 10⁹/l, serum iron 18.8 μmol/l, TIBC 45.0 μmol/l, bilirubin 20 μmol/l, aspartate transaminase 40 U/l, alkaline phosphatase 98 U/l, urea 8.3 mmol/l, plasma sodium 140 mmol/l, potassium 3.7 mmol/l, WR positive, Treponema immobilization test negative, ANF negative, proteins 72 g/l, albumin 39 g/l, MSU sterile, urobilinogen positive, haemoglobin negative.

1. What are the two most likely reasons for her vertebral collapse?
2. What are the four most useful investigations to define the cause of her anaemia?

This woman might have collapsed her vertebrae through **steroid enhanced osteoporosis** or **neoplastic deposits**.

The blood tests indicate that she has a haemolytic anaemia associated with a false positive WR. Her **peripheral blood** should be examined for signs of a microangiopathic picture with its grossly deformed red cells, and a **bone marrow aspiration** and **trephine** should be considered.

At this age her haemolytic anaemia must be acquired and in the absence of any significant drug history or chronic infection, one should look for associated antibodies. A **direct Coombs' test** should be carried out, to look for 'warm antibodies'. **Cold agglutinins** and **plasma electrophoresis** for abnormal proteins, which are ususally of IgM class, should be sought and the level of **haptoglobins** checked, a low level being compatible with intravascular haemolysis. **Ham's test for acid haemolysis** will identify the rare cases of paroxysmal nocturnal haemoglobinuria which is due to an acquired red cell defect.

The direct Coombs' test was positive in this patient. About 50% of patients with a haemolytic anaemia associated with warm antibodies have underlying disorders, either malignancies including lymphomas or connective tissue diseases.

The bone scan suggested more neoplastic deposits in the spine and the lesion at T10 was needle biopsied under X-ray control. This confirmed the diagnosis of neoplasia, and the patient unfortunately died of her ovarian carcinoma a few months later.

Case 76

A 32-year-old woman teacher presented with a three-month history of episodes of transient painless vertical diplopia. The double vision was worse on looking up and to the right, the attacks lasted for several hours and tended to happen more towards the end of the day. Apart from feeling more tired recently (which she ascribed to the imminence of the A level exams) she was otherwise well. Three years previously she had had a partial thyroidectomy for primary hyperthyroidism and since then had been taking 0.1 mg thyroxine daily.

On examination she had normal visual acuities. Her pupils were equal and the reflexes normal. There was partial ptosis of the right upper lid, the left was normal. Ocular movements of the right eye were limited in elevation, the left were full. Optic discs and visual fields were full. General examination was otherwise normal.

Investigations: Hb 11.2 g/dl, WBC 6.5 × 10⁹/l, ESR 15 mm/h. Urea 4.2 mmol/l, plasma sodium 137 mmol/l, plasma potassium 3.7 mmol/l, serum calcium 2.4 mmol/l, serum T4 slightly low, T3 normal, TSH normal. Skull and chest X-rays were normal.

1. What is the most likely diagnosis?
2. How would you confirm this?
3. If this was normal what other diagnosis would you consider?

This lady presents with transient vertical diplopia which is due to the inability to elevate her right eye, and a ptosis. In spite of her previous hyperthyroidism, thyroid eye disease is a most unlikely cause of her diplopia as it virtually never produces a ptosis.

In any transient or variable ptosis, **myasthenia gravis** must be considered, there is an association with thyroid disease and it is the most likely diagnosis in this patient. She should have a **tensilon test** which must be performed with caution as respiratory or cardiovascular collapse is unfortunately not uncommon following this test and nasty accidents do happen. Some authorities recommend observing the effect of a control injection of saline followed by a test dose of 1–2 mg of Tensilon. Acetyl choline receptor antibodies should be looked for as they are a reliable indicator of myasthenia gravis, although they can sometimes be negative when the myasthenia is limited to the ocular muscles. An EMG should show fatiguability; single fibre studies are helpful, but these require a stoical patient and are time consuming. Mediastinal tomography and CT scanning will indicate whether a thymoma is present; the presence of striated muscle antibodies is said to correlate with this.

Other causes of her diplopia include a **partial 3rd nerve palsy**; the absence of pain and pupillary involvement are against compression of the nerve from a posterior communicating artery aneurysm. The lesion in this patient would be isolated to the superior division of the third nerve and would probably be located in the superior ophthalmic fissure. Local orbital infiltrations or a sphenoidal ridge meningioma would be possible causes, although one might expect the patient to have some pain and proptosis from these. Skull X-ray and an orbital CT scan would show the lesion; sometimes inflammation from an infected frontal sinus can produce this picture. Familial ocular myopathies are usually symmetrical and the normality of the other eye excludes these conditions. The Eaton–Lambert syndrome never affects ocular muscles.

Treatment of myasthenia is with oral anticholinesterases, corticosteroids and azathioprine; plasmapheresis is useful in acute exacerbations. Thymectomy is indicated in the presence of thymic hyperplasia or thymoma.

Case 77

A 30-year-old woman was referred for a physician's opinion by the local optician. She had gone there for a new pair of glasses as she thought that eyestrain was responsible for her recent headaches. At that time she was found to have marked optic disc swelling in her left eye and a suspicion of this in the right. Past medical history was unremarkable, but for the past two years she had been seeing a psychiatrist for depression and marital problems. Her periods were somewhat irregular and she had recently put on weight. She was on no medication and neither drank nor smoked.

On examination, her blood pressure was 140/90 mmHg. There were no abnormal physical findings apart from her obesity and optic disc swelling. Her visual acuity and fields were normal (apart from enlarged blind spots). She was depressed and was convinced that she was going to die.

1. How would you confirm that the right optic disc was swollen?
2. What is the most likely diagnosis?
3. Suggest the three most useful investigations in reaching the diagnosis.

Optic discs can be swollen from many causes and these days papilloedema implies swelling from raised CSF pressure. Confirmation that this patient has bilateral papilloedema is readily and simply shown by **fluorescein angiography** of the fundus—the suspected optic disc will leak dye if it is swollen. Many patients might be spared unnecessary and dangerous investigations by this simple test.

In a young person who has an unremarkable history together with essentially normal physical findings apart from obesity and papilloedema, some evidence of endocrine imbalance and a normal blood pressure, **benign intracranial hypertension** must be the most likely diagnosis. However, this is a diagnosis of exclusion requiring full investigation to exclude a space-occupying lesion or obstructive hydrocephalus. The essential investigations are a **skull X-ray** and a **computerized axial tomographic scan**. If the CT scan is normal with small or normal sized ventricles, a **lumbar puncture** should be performed to measure pressure and confirm that the cytology and biochemistry of the CSF is normal. Bilateral carotid angiography is only indicated if a mass lesion is shown on scanning and air encephalography has been superseded by CT scanning. A **serum calcium** and **serology for syphilis** would be useful.

The CSF pressure can usually be controlled by carbonic anhydrase inhibitors, e.g. acetazolamide, but repeated lumbar punctures are sometimes used. The most serious complication of benign intracranial hypertension is progressive visual failure due to chronic unrelieved papilloedema and decompression of the optic nerves or lumbar-peritoneal shunting is then required.

Benign intracranial hypertension can be associated with a variety of conditions namely obesity, the oral contraceptive pill, steroid treatment or withdrawal, middle ear disease, head trauma, hypervitaminosis A and hypocalcaemia. The condition has also been recorded following the use of nalidixic acid, nitrofurantoin and tetracyclines.

Case 78

A 64-year-old woman had the following past history. She had developed rheumatic fever after her first pregnancy when she was 25. She was rested in bed for three months, treated with aspirin, and made a good recovery. Six years later, during her second pregnancy, she became dyspnoeic on exertion, developed cardiac failure and recurrent small haemoptyses. Four years later, when she was 35, she had sudden onset of pain in both legs which became white, cold and pale. The condition improved over the next 36 hours. The following year she had three attacks of pneumonia and a bowel resection for a mesenteric embolus. Histology showed a normal thrombus. When the patient was 41, she had a mitral valvotomy to relieve her orthopnoea and dyspnoea on minimal exertion and after this she was able to walk two miles. She remained well but developed the murmurs of mitral and tricuspid incompetence as well as her mitral stenosis. When she was 60 she had an episode of severe central chest pain in bed lasting five hours. She was anticoagulated but two months later she had an episode of left loin pain and frank haematuria. Anticoagulants were stopped.

1. What was the most likely cause of haemoptysis in the second pregnancy?
2. What was the cause of her leg symptoms when she was 35?
3. What are the three most likely causes of her chest pain when she was 60?
4. What are the two most likely causes of the haematuria?
5. What are the likely ECG abnormalities this patient would show before her episode of chest pain four years ago?

There are four reasons why haemoptyses may occur more commonly in patients with mitral stenosis:

1. **Venous engorgement occurs in the pulmonary vascular bed** as a consequence of the high left atrial pressure. These veins may rupture causing haemoptysis. Pathologically haemosiderin is deposited in the lungs causing mottling on the chest X-ray and which may eventually calcify.
2. **Pulmonary oedema** may occur with the expectoration of blood stained frothy sputum.
3. **Pulmonary emboli** are more frequent, presumably due to decreased cardiac output and less active lifestyles of the patients.
4. There is an increased incidence of **chest infections**.

In addition, the patient may have an increased bleeding tendency through the use of **anticoagulants**. In this patient the most likely cause of her early haemoptyses would be her pulmonary venous engorgement.

Embolization may occur at any stage of her disease, but especially after the onset of atrial fibrillation, which often marks an increase in the patient's deterioration. This woman has a **saddle embolus blocking the bifurcation of the aorta**. If a patient presents with embolization requiring surgical removal, then the embolus must be sent for histology to exclude a left atrial myxoma which may give identical cardiac signs. Embolization must also raise the possibility of infective endocarditis, although this is a rare complication of pure mitral stenosis.

Her chest pain at the age of 60 might have been due to **pulmonary embolism** or a **myocardial infarction**. The latter may be due to a **coronary embolus** as well as secondary to atheroma.

Her haematuria may well have resulted from **over-anticoagulation** or from a **renal embolus**.

In the ECG, the earliest sign is that of P mitrale if the patient is in sinus rhythm. This, of course, disappears with the onset of atrial fibrillation. As the mitral stenosis advances, there may be changes of **right ventricular hypertrophy** and **right axis deviation**.

Case 79

A 20-year-old girl was admitted to hospital in a state of collapse with a history of malaise and lethargy for two days associated with vomiting. On the day of admission she complained of a severe headache and weakness. She had become confused and disoriented and vomited profusely.

Examination showed delirium, dehydration, a tachycardia of 140 per minute, blood pressure of 110/60 mmHg, temperature 36°C. Purpuric areas were identified on the arms. There was neck stiffness, a positive Kernig's sign and signs of cerebral irritability. The optic discs were pink with early papilloedema. Reflexes were normal and the plantar response showed a marked withdrawal reaction. The right knee joint was swollen, hot and tender.

Investigations: Hb 13 g/dl, WBC 25 × 10^9/l, neutrophils 19.7 × 10^9/l, platelets 20 × 10^9/l, plasma sodium 137 mmol/l, potassium 3.4 mmol/l, bicarbonate 16 mmol/l, urea 18.2 mmol/l. CSF: pressure raised. WBC 3.5 × 10^9/l, polymorphs 100%. RBC 1.2 × 10^9/l. No organisms seen. Protein 0.8 g/l. Sugar less than 0.25 mmol/l.

1. What would be your initial therapy?
2. What agent do you suspect is responsible for her meningitis?
3. What complication do you suspect might be present?
4. What would be the two most useful tests to confirm this?
5. Give two possible causes for her swollen right knee.

This girl is seriously ill with meningitis and the clinical picture and CSF findings indicate a bacterial infection. Although the organisms were not identified on initial gram stains of the spinal fluid, the most likely causative agent in this case is the **Meningococcus**. However, infection with pneumococcus or *Haemophilus influenzae* must be considered.

General treatment consists of the correction of fluid and electrolyte deficits, adequate oxygenation and maintenance of cardiovascular function. Specific antibiotic regimes vary but drugs should be started immediately in high doses and intravenously. They should cover all likely organisms and suggested regimes are **benzylpenicillin** and **chloramphenicol** (with or without a sulphonamide) or **ampicillin**. Many strains of the Meningococcus are now resistant to sulphonamides and ampicillin resistant Haemophilus strains are now present, especially in the USA.

Although the meningococcaemia may be associated with many skin manifestations including rose spots, petechiae and frank purpura, the co-existence of severe thrombocytopenia and bruising suggests the possibility of **disseminated intravascular coagulation**, which should be investigated by **clotting studies** and examination of the serum for **fibrinogen degradation products**. It may be necessary to correct the clotting abnormalities by the use of blood products and some would give heparin in an attempt to stop the coagulation although there is no evidence that it improves the outcome in such cases.

Acute cerebral oedema may be life-threatening and require treatment with mannitol or dexamethasone. Some would also give steroid therapy to the seriously ill patient with no evidence of cerebral oedema, especially in view of the possibility of haemorrhage into the adrenal glands. Again there is no definite evidence of benefit. **Seizures** are common and are treated conventionally.

The swollen right knee could reflect a **pyogenic arthritis**, consequent upon septicaemia, but the possibility of a **haemarthrosis** should be entertained, although this is an unusual manifestation of disseminated intravascular coagulation. A sterile polyarthropathy may be found in meningococcal infections, although this usually occurs in conjunction with a chronic meningococcaemia.

Polyvalent vaccines are available against some strains of Meningococci.

Case 80

A 65-year-old woman was admitted as a surgical emergency with a four day history of vomiting, diarrhoea and upper abdominal pain. She had previously been well except for recent weight loss and lethargy.

On examination she was dark skinned, but pale, and had patches of vitiligo. She was dehydrated, shocked, her pulse rapid and weak and she had generalized abdominal tenderness.

Initial investigations showed: Hb 14.5 g/dl, WBC 18 × 10⁹/l, plasma sodium 137 mmol/l, potassium 8.8 mmol/l, chloride 100 mmol/l, bicarbonate 8 mmol/l, blood sugar 33.3 mmol/l, urea 32.2 mmol/l, amylase normal. Chest X-ray (erect and supine) showed no evidence of gas under the diaphragm. The ECG revealed peaked T-waves, but no evidence of infarction. Abdominal X-ray unremarkable.

Initial treatment was rehydration, insulin, antibiotics and hydrocortisone and she improved gradually. Three days later while continuing to improve on a carbohydrate restricted diet, oral fluids and insulin, she remained hypotensive.

Investigations at this time revealed plasma sodium 124 mmol/l, potassium 4.1 mmol/l, chloride 101 mmol/l, bicarbonate 19.7 mmol/l, blood sugar 8.6 mmol/l, urea 23.5 mmol/l.

1. From what four conditions does this patient suffer?
2. What would be the three most useful investigations on recovery?

At the time of admission this woman was referred to the surgical team with a provisional diagnosis of a perforated peptic ulcer or acute pancreatitis, neither of which were borne out by subsequent investigations. She had undoubted **diabetic ketoacidosis** with gross dehydration and renal failure. Diabetic ketoacidosis is frequently precipitated by an underlying infection or a myocardial infarction, and here an infection was thought to be the likely cause, though no primary focus was apparent. She was thought to be septicaemic with shock and she was treated with broad spectrum antibiotics and steroids.

The combination of pigmentation, vitiligo and hypotension, associated with a previous history of abdominal pain is strongly suggestive of Addison's disease. The subsequent finding of hyponatraemia supports this concept. Therefore, the most likely explanation of the initial presentation is that she had **diabetic ketoacidosis, Addisonian crisis, renal failure** with possibly a marked pre-renal element and **septicaemia**, and the fortuitous administration of hydrocortisone initially masked the Addisonian component.

Further investigations should include assessment of adrenal function. The patient should be treated with **dexamethasone** and a **synacthen stimulation test** should be performed to assess adrenal responsiveness and **adrenal antibodies** should be sought. Once fully replaced with steroids, the renal function should be assessed by doing a **creatinine clearance** to see the degree, if any, of primary renal disease.

The association of Addison's disease and diabetes mellitus is well recognized.

Case 81

A 28-year-old woman attended her general practitioner three times in a two-month period with vaginal Candidiasis. On each ocasion, the GP prescribed treatment with clotrimazole which both she and her boyfriend used correctly.

She returned with a sore throat and pain on swallowing solids. Her GP noted pharyngitis and biltateral enlarged, tender cervical lymph nodes. He arranged some blood tests, which showed: Hb 10.7 g/dl, WBC 3.2 × 10⁹/l, platelets 220 × 10⁹/l, Paul–Bunnell test negative, fasting glucose normal.

An outpatient appointment with a haematologist was arranged, but before this could take place, the patient was taken to casualty by her boyfriend. She had developed a non-productive cough of ten days duration, followed by three days of dyspnoea which had worsened despite oral amoxycillin and erythromycin.

On examination, her temperature was 38.2°C, and she was deeply cyanosed. She had oral candidiasis. Respiratory rate 30/min, pulse 120/min regular, BP 110/70 mmHg. Her venous pressure was not raised, and heart sounds were normal. Examination of the chest was normal, as were abdominal and nervous systems.

Investigations: Hb 9.8 g/dl, WBC 5.4 × 10⁹/l, 93% neutrophils, platelets 243 × 10⁹/l. Urea and electrolytes and liver function tests normal. ECG showed sinus tachycardia with incomplete right bundle branch block. Chest X-ray showed bilateral soft basal and midzone shadows of a reticular pattern. Arterial blood gases on air: PaO_2 6.1 kPa (46 mmHg), $PaCO_2$ 3.5 kPa (26 mmHg), pH 7.50.

1. What is the most likely diagnosis?
2. Suggest four useful investigations.
3. What is the treatment?
4. Why did she have pain on swallowing?

This young woman has suffered recurrent vaginal Candida infections, despite adequate treatment, and is not diabetic. She developed pain on swallowing and lymphadenopathy and was found to be leucopenic; she now has a normal total white cell count, but the cells are almost exclusively made up of neutrophils. She has oral candidiasis, which could be the consequence of antibiotic therapy, and a syndrome of cyanosis, tachypnoea, a clear chest on auscultation and widespread radiological shadowing. These features taken all together strongly suggest an 'atypical pneumonia', particularly *Pneumocystis carinii* pneumonia (PCP) in a woman with impaired cell-mediated immunity. Other pneumonias such as **viral, candidal** or **fungal** are possible, as are **Legionella** or **Mycoplasma**, although some response to erythromycin would be expected.

The possible underlying disorder includes **acquired immunodeficiency syndrome**, due to chronic infection with **human immunodeficiency virus** (**HIV**). This affects heterosexual women as well as men. **Anti-HIV antibodies** should be checked after counselling; in this case, these were present. Other causes of impaired cell-mediated immunity include **lymphoproliferative** disorders and some **myeloproliferative** diseases.

Further investigations should include **blood film**, acute and convalescent **viral titres, Legionella** and **Mycoplasma serology, culture** of **blood, throat** and **urine** and if anti-HIV negative, **bone marrow aspiration** and **lymph node biopsy**.

The diagnosis of PCP depends upon demonstation of the organism. **Sputum induction** using nebulized hypertonic saline followed by silver staining provides the diagnosis in many cases. When negative, **bronchoscopy with lavage** and/or **transbronchial biopsy** may be necessary. Treatment ideally is with high-dose intravenous **co-trimoxazole. Pentamidine** is an alternative although this produces a slower response and is more toxic. Good evidence supports the concurrent use of **glucocorticoids**. Nebulized pentamidine once weekly or daily low-dose (960 mg) co-trimoxazole are effective secondary prophylaxis.

Pain on swallowing (odynophagia) may be due in this case to oesophageal infection with Candida, herpes simplex or cytomegalovirus.

Case 82

A 79-year-old woman was referred from the eye clinic. She had presented complaining of floaters in her vision and was found to have the fundal appearance of retinal vein obstruction.

She said she had been short of breath for a month after walking twenty or thirty yards and felt too weak to do her housework. She lived in a ground floor flat. Her appetite was poor and she had lost about a stone in weight over the previous three months. Direct questioning revealed that she had had frequent recent nose bleeds and that her fingers became white in cold weather.

On examination she was plethoric. She had a regular pulse of 80, blood pressure 140/100 mmHg with an ejection systolic murmur at the apex. She could lie flat with no dyspnoea. In her abdomen the liver was palpable 2 cm and spleen 3 cm. There was no lymphadenopathy and apart from the fundal appearances examination was otherwise normal.

1. From this history alone what are the three most likely diagnoses?

In outpatients, blood examination showed Hb 8.7 g/dl, MCHC 30 g/dl, MCH 30 fl, platelets $109 \times 10^9//l$, ESR 260 (calculated), film-rouleaux and plasma cells. Later the MSU, urea and electrolytes, calcium, phosphate and hepatic enzymes were found to be normal.

2. Suggest three possible complications of the most likely diagnosis that this patient may have.
3. What would be your urgent management?
4. What would be the three most relevant investigations?

This woman has a mild malaise associated with hepatosplenomegaly. From her history the diagnosis lay between **Waldenstrom's macroglobulinaemia**, a **lymphoma** and **polycythaemia rubra vera** which would be unusual at this age. Myeloma would be unlikely with the absence of bone pain with liver and spleen involvement.

Patients with macroglobulinaemia may develop a **hyperviscosity** syndrome due to their high levels of plasma globulins. This is thought to cause the fundal appearances, malaise and sometimes neurological sequelae resulting from cerebral thromboses. **Bleeding episodes** are common due to plasma protein, clotting factor and platelet interactions and her **Raynaud's phenomenon** is probably due to cryoglobulins. Occasionally **amyloidosis** may involve the parenchymal organs.

This patient's hyperviscosity threatens her vision and she requires urgent **plasmapharesis** to remove the excess protein from her blood.

To establish a diagnosis a **bone marrow, plasma protein** estimation and **immunopharesis** are necessary. Her globulin level was 90 g/l (9 g%) with the abnormal protein confined to the IgM band.

Case 83

A 25-year-old housewife was brought to casualty by her sister. She had found her to be drowsy when she visited her that morning, and she had vomited three times. She had been perfectly well the previous evening and had no relevant past medical history. Her children aged 2 and 4 and her husband were well, although he had lost his job as a lorry driver following a series of seizures which were felt to be alcohol-related. She took no medications other than the oral contraceptive pill, smoked 20 cigarettes daily and drank five pints of lager a week.

On examination she was afebrile with no meningism or photophobia. The abnormalities were confined to the nervous sytem. She was drowsy and disorientated. She had coarse nystagmus in all directions of gaze with a vertical component. Fundoscopy was normal, as were the cranial nerves otherwise. Tone, power, sensation and reflexes were normal in the limbs and both plantars were downgoing. She had a broad-based gait and bilateral poor finger–nose and heel–shin co-ordination.

Investigations: urea and electrolytes, full blood count, clotting, liver function tests and amylase all normal. Blood ethanol undetectable. Contrast-enhanced computerized tomograph (CT scan) of the brain was normal. Examination of the cerebrospinal fluid was normal.

1. Suggest four possible diagnoses.
2. What is the most likely diagnosis?
3. What is the single most useful further investigation?

This young woman presents with diminished consciousness, bilateral cerebellar signs and vertical nystagmus. She is afebrile with no meningism, and the CSF is normal, making a diagnosis of **meningitis** or **encephalitis** less likely. Vertical nystagmus suggests a brainstem localization and **brainstem demyelination**, **vascular malformation** or **tumour** are possibilities. A contrasted CT brain scan does not exclude these diagnoses as the posterior fossa is often poorly seen; magnetic resonance imaging (MRI) is more effective.

The combination of an encephalopathy with the brainstem and cerebellar features, however, make a **metabolic aetiology** most likely. An overdose of her husband's **anticonvulsant medications** is a unifying diagnosis. Phenytoin and carbamazepine can cause these features, and may provoke seizures when present in toxic levels. The most useful further investigation is an urgent **blood** and **urine drug screen**.

Wernicke's encephalopathy may cause a similar picture due to thiamine deficiency, particularly in alcoholics. Red blood cell transketolase activity can be assayed in vitro but the result often takes some time. The response to thiamine replacement is often dramatic.

Case 84

A 61-year-old printer presented with a month's history of abdominal distension and some weight loss. He mentioned his gait was funny; he felt as if his right leg flapped but he could feel the ground. He smoked 40 cigarettes a day, had a cough and some shortness of breath on exertion. He said he drank several pints of beer a day.

On examination he was thin and slightly jaundiced. He had several spider naevi and palmar erythema and a Dupuytren's contracture. There was ascites and a palpable liver 6 cm below the costal margin. Neurologically the only findings were a slight tremor and signs in his lower limbs. There was wasting of both calves together with some fasciculation. There was weakness of dorsiflexion and eversion of both feet, more marked on the right. The right ankle jerk was absent and the plantar responses were flexor. There was a slight reduction of sensation to touch and vibration in both legs.

Investigations showed: Hb 12.4 g/dl, MCV 110 fl. Target cells in film. WBC 8 × 10⁹/l. ESR 35 mm/h, bilirubin 113μ mol/l, alkaline phosphatase 210 U/l, aspartate transaminase 45 U/l, albumin 26 g/l, α-fetoprotein—negative. Chest X-ray report; 'High diaphragms with some collapse at the left base—probably due to ascites'. Barium swallow, meal and enema normal. Liver scan—enlarged liver, patchy diffuse uptake of isotope. Liver biopsy—alcoholic cirrhosis with fatty changes. Lumbar spine X-rays normal.

1. What type of lesion, and at what site, would account for the motor symptoms in the right leg?
2. What are the four most likely causes of this?
3. What would be the two most useful investigations at this stage?

This man has the classical signs of a lower motor neurone lesion, namely weakness and wasting of muscles with absent reflexes. The peronei and extensors of the foot are supplied by L4, L5 and S1 and hence these nerves must be affected somewhere along their course from anterior horn cell to muscle. The concomitant sensory changes suggest the lesion is a **peripheral neuropathy**.

Other significant features in his history are his weight loss, heavy smoking and drinking, together with signs of cirrhosis and ascites. Of interest in his peripheral neuropathy is the preponderance of motor over sensory signs.

Alcoholic neuropathy must be considered but it is usually painful with marked hypersensitivity to light touch. Motor neuropathies are typical of **porphyria** or **lead toxicity** which might be relevant to his job as a printer. A motor neuropathy also occurs following infection (**Guillain–Barré syndrome** or, rarely now, with **diphtheria** but there is nothing in the history to suggest this).

Taking into account the other features of the case, the most appropriate diagnosis would be **carcinomatous neuropathy**, which typically gives both motor and sensory changes. In more than half the cases this is a non-metastatic complication of a bronchial carcinoma although sporadic cases occur with a variety of other malignant disease, including lymphoma. It may occur without any other suggestion of malignant disease and hence prompt and thorough investigation is necessary. We were temporarily distracted by the chest X-ray report but **bronchoscopy** and **sputum cytology** confirmed the presence of an oat cell carcinoma and laparoscopy visualized hepatic and peritoneal secondary deposits that were no doubt contributing to his ascites.

Diabetes mellitus and vitamin B12 deficiency both tend to produce a symmetrical sensory neuropathy and were rapidly excluded by biochemical tests. His macrocytosis was a manifestation of his high alcohol intake. There was no family history with this man to suggest any of the inherited causes of neuropathy.

Case 85

A 25-year-old previously well bodybuilder presented to casualty with severe breathlessness. This had progressed over a two-week period, and followed a brief flu-like illness associated with sore throat, myalgia and runny nose. These symptoms had resolved. The level of breathlessness was now such that he was unable to walk more than five metres on the flat, having been previously unlimited. There was no cough, wheeze or chest pain. He took no medications and denied the use of anabolic steroids. No relevant medical or family history.

On examination he looked unwell. He had an oral temperature of 37.4°C, pulse 110 per minute regular, blood pressure 90/60 mmHg lying and standing, no paradox. His venous pressure was 7 cm above the sternal angle, falling with inspiration. Respiratory rate 24 per minute. Chest expansion was good and equal and percussion note resonant. There were fine bibasal inspiratory crackles and no wheeze. There was a soft apical third heart sound and no murmurs. There was no peripheral oedema. Examination of the abdominal and nervous systems was unremarkable.

Investigations in casualty: Hb 14.3 g/dl, WBC 14 × 10⁹/l, platelets 280 × 10⁹/l, sodium 140 mmol/l, potassium 3.7 mmol/l, urea 6.7 mmol/l. ECG showed sinus tachycardia at a rate of 110/min with T-wave inversion in leads V1–V6, I, II, and III. There were frequent multifocal ventricular ectopics. Arterial blood gases on air: PO_2 10.2 kPa (77 mmHg), PCO_2 2.9 kPa (22 mmHg), pH 7.47. Urine dipstick and microscopy normal.

While waiting for a chest X-ray, he suffered a cardiac arrest and the ECG monitor showed ventricular tachycardia. He returned to sinus rhythm after a 360 J DC shock but had two further episodes of ventricular fibrillation before being resuscitated and admitted to the intensive care unit.

1. What is the diagnosis?
2. Suggest three further useful investigations.
3. Suggest six important features in his management.

The history of a viral illness followed by progressive severe breathlessness with physical signs of heart failure and rhythm disturbance suggest a diagnosis of **viral myocarditis**. An underlying **cardiomyopathy** is a possibility but less likely with this presentation. Although a third heart sound may be a normal finding in a healthy young person, in combination with a raised venous pressure, resting tachycardia, bibasal crackles in the chest and hypotension, it is probably pathological. The ECG abnormalities are consistent with myocarditis. There is no strong evidence for cardiac tamponade which would be more likely in the presence of pulsus paradoxus and a prominent 'X' descent of the JVP. A rise in the venous pressure during inspiration (Kussmaul's sign) is uncommon.

Further investigations include **echocardiogram** to assess left and right ventricular systolic function, valve function and to examine for pericardial effusion. Tamponade is a clinical not echocardiographic diagnosis, but it may be suggested by diastolic collapse of the right ventricle. In this case, the ventricles were dilated with globally severely impaired function with no effusion. Blood should be taken for **viral antibody titres** in the acute and convalescent phase. A definitive aetiology is often not found, but Coxsackie, influenza and Epstein–Barr virus are implicated in some cases. **Cardiac enzymes** such as creatine phosphokinase and hydroxybutyrate dehydrogenase may be greatly elevated. **Endomyocardial biopsy** performed during cardiac catherization will show acute inflammatory changes and confirm the diagnosis.

Management in this case should aim at stabilization of cardiac rhythm and treatment of heart failure and of the underlying myocarditis. **Intravenous lignocaine** and **correction of hypokalaemia** are important initially, in view of recurrent ventricular fibrillation, although **amiodarone** may be given to prevent further malignant dysrhythmias. **Oxygen, intravenous diuretics** and **opiates** should be given to treat heart failure, and **inotropic support** with agents such as dopamine and dobutamine may be necessary if there is evidence of end organ damage due to under-perfusion (e.g. poor urine output or rising urea). In the longer term, an **angiotensin-converting enzyme inhibitor** should be given. There is no convincing evidence that treatment with steroids or other immunosuppressants improves outcome.

The majority of cases of viral myocarditis recover. Some cases, however, result in chronic heart failure and **cardiac transplantation** may be indicated.

Case 86

A 14-year-old boy was taken to his general practitioner having been unwell for one week. His symptoms included swinging fever, up to 39°C, cough and runny nose, aching joints and diarrhoea. His GP noted a flushed appearance, conjunctival congestion, and redness of the palms and soles. There was a pharyngitis and the boy's tongue looked particularly red. There was tender cervical lymphadenopathy but no hepatosplenomegaly. The remainder of the examination was unremarkable. The GP diagnosed a viral respiratory infection, and suggested a high fluid intake and paracetamol; he did not prescribe antibiotics but asked to see the boy again if the symptoms did not resolve.

Four weeks later, the GP was called to the boy's home. While playing football, he had developed severe pain in the centre of the chest and had vomited twice.

Examination showed an afebrile, frightened boy with a tachycardia, rate 130/min regular, blood pressure 90/60 mmHg. There was desquamation of the palms and soles. There was a soft apical ejection systolic murmur and a gallop rhythm. There was no other abnormality.

The GP arranged for the boy to be seen in casualty where the following investigations were obtained: Hb 11.3 g/dl, WBC 14 × 10⁹/l, platelets 478 × 10⁹/l, ESR 65 mm/h. Blood film, urea and electrolytes, random glucose, and chest X-ray normal. Paul–Bunnell test negative. An ECG showed sinus rhythm with 4 mm ST segment elevation in leads II, III and aVf, and Q-waves in the same leads.

1. What is the diagnosis?
2. What treatments may have prevented this complication?
3. Suggest two further useful investigations.
4. What treatment should this boy receive now?

This young boy has presented with a history and ECG changes diagnostic of acute inferior myocardial infarction. This is an extremely unusual diagnosis in a boy of 14 years, and causes other than coronary atheroma, such as an arteritis, should be considered. In view of this history, **Kawasaki syndrome** is the most likely diagnosis. This is a systemic vasculitis of unknown aetiology. It occurs predominantly in Japan, where the incidence is 15/100 000/year usually in children under the age of 4, and where almost 100 000 cases have occurred since its description in 1967. It is however reported increasingly worldwide in children and young adults of all ethnic descent. The diagnosis is made clinically on the basis of fever, red palms and soles with subsequent desquamation, conjunctival congestion, red lips, 'strawberry tongue', a polymorphous exanthema and lymphadenopathy. Investigations show a raised ESR and C-reactive protein, thrombocytosis, leukocytosis and anaemia.

Medium-sized arteries, including coronary arteries are affected most frequently. 20–30% develop cardiac complications. This may be evident as acute myocarditis, but coronary artery aneurysms occur in up to 40% of cases, thrombosis or rupture of which may cause myocardial infarction.

There is evidence from randomized prospective trials that treatment with high-dose intravenous **gamma-globulins** in the acute phase reduces the cardiovascular complications. **Aspirin** also protects, although the optimal dose and protective mechanism is unclear.

Further investigations should include **echocardiography** to assess ventricular function and may show aneurysms, and **coronary arteriography**. Experience in Japan suggests that acute myocardial infarction should be dealt with in conventional ways, with the use of **thrombolysis** and **aspirin**. **Coronary artery bypass grafting** has been carried out. Rhythm disturbances and heart failure may occur and **transplantation** may be necessary.

Myocardial infarction in the young may also be due to coronary artery spasm due to cocaine abuse, and traumatic thrombosis or rupture of coronary arteries has been reported in rugby players or following road accidents, but there is no suggestion of these causes in this history.

Case 87

A 45-year-old bricklayer was admitted to hospital with a history of increasing dyspnoea over the previous four days. There was no history of chest pain, cough or haemoptysis. He had no previous illnesses and was on no medication. His mother had maturity onset diabetes.

On examination, he was not breathless at rest, but was slightly cyanosed. Blood pressure was 160/105 mmHg, radial pulse was 126 per minute and irregular, and of poor volume. His JVP was raised 2 cm and heart sounds were normal. In the chest there were fine inspiratory crepitations at both bases, and in the abdomen, the liver was palpable one finger's breadth below the costal margin. ECG showed atrial fibrillation with T-wave inversion at leads V4-V6. Chest X-ray on admission showed cardiomegaly and pulmonary oedema.

The patient was treated with diuretics and oxygen. Cardioversion was unsuccessful, even using 400 joules. He was digitalized and on his other treatment his pulmonary oedema cleared, and his blood pressure settled to 140/90 mmHg. Serial chest X-rays showed gradual reduction in heart size.

Investigations showed: Hb 13.2 g/dl, MCV 100 fl, WBC 9.3 × 10^9/l, platelets 286 × 10^9/l. Urea and electrolytes, glucose tolerance test and thyroid function tests were all normal. Viral titres showed no evidence of recent infection. Cholesterol 1.7 mmol/l and triglycerides 10.6 mmol/l.

Echocardiography showed that the left atrium and both ventricles were enlarged. The mitral and aortic valves were normal. The left ventricle contracted poorly with an ejection fraction of 30%.

1. What is the likely diagnosis?

The patient has biventricular failure with atrial fibrillation. The ventricular rate is not fast enough to tip a normal heart into failure. In this case, his atrial fibrillation is due to neither thyrotoxicosis nor mitral valve disease. There is nothing in the history to suggest ischaemic heart disease, nor a recent infection either viral myocarditis or a bacterial pneumonia, both of which may precipitate atrial fibrillation.

There are several important pointers in this man's investigations, namely macrocytosis and hypertriglyceridaemia. The latter is commonly due to diabetes but the patient has a normal glucose tolerance test. These features, plus evidence on the echocardiogram, makes a diagnosis of **alcoholic cardiomyopathy** most likely. This condition often presents with arrhythmias, particularly atrial fibrillation. The findings of poorly contracting left ventricle and three chamber enlargement are not specific for alcohol, but indicate a congestive cardiomyopathy. Alcohol may affect the heart in several ways: apart from cobalt poisoning, and a congestive cardiomyopathy, the patient may develop thiamine deficiency (beri-beri) which clinically presents with high output cardiac failure.

Case 88

A 76-year-old woman was referred to outpatients with a six-month history of lethargy, anorexia and fevers. Her family were concerned that she was continuing to lose weight, and her daughter, a nursing sister, had measured temperatures varying between 37.5°C and 38.5°C in the month leading to referral. There had been no change in bowel habit, no dysuria or cough. Her husband had been well and they had both visited Malta three months before her illness began, but she had not felt well enough to travel abroad this year. She was a non-smoker, and drank small quantities of sherry infrequently. She had a cholecystectomy 15 years previously. She took no medications.

On examination she looked unwell and had clearly lost weight. Temperature 37.3°C, pulse 100 regular, blood pressure 150/80 mm Hg. She was clinically euthyroid and the remainder of the examination was unremarkable. She was admitted for investigation. Her temperature continued to vary in the fashion described by her daughter.

Results of investigations: Hb 9.0 g/dl, WBC 13 × 10⁹/l (normal differential), platelets 620 × 10⁹/l, ESR 85 mm/hour, sodium 143 mmol/l, potassium 4.5 mmol/l, urea 6.1 mmol/l, bilirubin 20 μmol/l, alkaline phosphatase 290 IU/l, AST 28 IU/l, albumin 34 g/l, globulins 42 g/l. Serum electrophoresis showed a polyclonal increase in gamma globulins with no oligoclonal band. Antinuclear factor (ANF) and antineutrophil cytoplasmic antibody (ANCA) each weakly positive, anti-DNA antibodies and rheumatoid factor negative. Urine microscopy normal and no Bence–Jones protein detected. Urine culture and six blood culture sets sterile. Brucella serology and viral titres including HIV negative. Chest X-ray and ECG normal. Tuberculin test negative at 1000 units. Upper gastrointestinal endoscopy, barium enema, IVP, abdominal ultrasound and abdominal CT scan all normal. Liver biopsy normal, bone marrow normal with negative staining and culture for Mycobacteria.

1. What is the likeliest diagnosis that has been overlooked in this lady?
2. What is the investigation of choice?
3. What is the appropriate treatment?

This unfortunate lady presents with a pyrexia of unknown origin (PUO) and has associated lethargy, anorexia and weight loss. She has been subject to a large number of investigations, none of which have given the answer.

Depending upon the definition used and the series examined, PUOs tend to fall into the following final diagnostic categories. Approximate frequencies from two large series are given, although a significant proportion are never diagnosed:

Infections	36–69%
Neoplasms	6–19%
Connective tissue diseases	3–13%
Other causes (e.g. drug fever, factitious fever)	

The more common causes are excluded by the investigations given. Note that a negative tuberculin test does not exclude tuberculosis, and in up to 10% of cases with disseminated disease the test is negative. There is however no other clinical evidence for tuberculosis and the bone marrow culture is negative. Renal carcinoma can present with a PUO but the urine, IVP and abdominal CT scan are all normal.

In this genuine case, further investigations were under consideration and included exploratory laparotomy and therapeutic trial of antituberculous chemotherapy or corticosteroids. The lady then developed frontal headaches, almost seven months after the onset of fevers. A **temporal artery biopsy** revealed **giant cell arteritis** and she made a dramatic response to high-dose **corticosteroids**, with resolution of the fever and weight gain. At no point during her illness did she have temporal artery or muscle tenderness.

A weakly positive ANF and ANCA are not uncommon in connective tissue diseases such as giant cell arteritis.

Case 89

A 30-year-old school teacher presented with a history of increasing dyspnoea over the previous six days. For the past two years she had had four or five episodes of nocturnal cough, sputum and dyspnoea which usually followed an upper respiratory tract infection. These episodes resolved over a week with a course of antibiotics. Her only other problem was dysmenorrhoea for which she took the oral contraceptive pill. On this occasion she failed to respond and developed a sharp short-lived right lower chest pain.

On examination, her temperature was 37.5°C. She was not cyanosed and her blood pressure was 130/80 mmHg; pulse 100 beats per minute, sinus rhythm. In the chest there were bilateral expiratory and inspiratory rhonchi and a few crepitations at the right base, but no rub. The abdomen, legs and central nervous system were all normal.

Investigations showed: Hb 12.8 g/dl, WBC 9.6 × 10^9 /l. Sputum culture was sterile. ESR was 25 mm/h. Chest X-ray showed some soft shadowing at the right base.

Her penicillin was changed to tetracycline and she was given bronchodilator tablets. A week later she felt considerably better and, although she continued to expectorate a little mucoid sputum, she was well enough to return to work. However, one month later she had a further episode of dyspnoea and on this occasion had coughed up a few flecks of blood mixed with some sputum.

On examination she was slightly breathless with evidence of mild bronchospasm. There were no other abnormal physical signs.

Chest X-ray showed resolution of the right lower zone changes, but newer shadowing at the left apex with the suggestion of some ring shadows was noted. ECG was normal. A ventilation/perfusion lung scan showed no evidence of pulmonary emboli.

1. What is the diagnosis?
2. Give three helpful investigations.

The patient gives a history of episodic dyspnoea often precipitated by upper respiratory tract infection. The physical findings are predominantly those of bronchospasm and in a previously fit, non-smoking patient, bronchial asthma is by far the most likely cause. This, however, has been complicated by an abnormal chest X-ray. The most common cause is bacterial infection and although sputum culture was sterile, the patient had had several days treatment with antibiotics. She does, however, develop some new X-ray changes and has a small haemoptysis. While this obviously raises the possibility of pulmonary emboli, this is unlikely without a perfusion defect with normal ventilation on lung scanning.

The appearance of transient pulmonary shadowing in an asthmatic is very suggestive of **allergic bronchopulmonary aspergillosis**. This is characteristically associated with **blood** and **sputum** eosinophilia and a **positive type 1 skin prick test to an extract of Aspergillus fumigatus**. Serum precipitins are less consistently present and culture of Aspergillus from the sputum is not universal. The concentration of immunoglobulin E (IgE) in the serum is usually raised but is non-specific.

Proximal bronchiectasis may occur at the site of previous infiltration and may explain the haemoptysis in this patient.

The disease is a potentially serious complication of extrinsic asthma and has been reported in as many as 20% of asthmatics admitted to hospital. It is a hypersensitivity reaction to *Aspergillus fumigatus* affecting bronchial walls and peripheral parts of the lung. The airway obstruction is often more than usually severe and there is a moderate reduction in gas transfer factor. Transient infiltration leaves permanent radiological change in half the patients and often leads to permanent functional impairment with bronchiectasis and lobar shrinkage. The diagnosis is important to make early as treatment with corticosteroids diminishes the frequency of acute attacks and reduces the likelihood of severe permanent lung damage.

Other causes of bronchospasm, fleeting shadows on a chest X-ray and eosinophilia include connective tissue diseases such as **Churg–Strauss** syndrome. Anti-neutrophil cytoplasmic antibodies (ANCA) should therefore be checked.

Case 90

A 38-year-old barman presented with a two day history of headache. This had been preceded by a short illness with myalgia, malaise and anorexia. Three years previously he had been hospitalized with an unexplained attack of abdominal pain, but which had settled after 36 hours of conservative treatment and had not recurred. He smoked 20 cigarettes a day and drank at least four pints of beer every night. His general practitioner had started him on penicillin three days prior to his admission.

On examination, his temperature was 38°C, blood pressure 130/76 mmHg, pulse 92 per minute and regular. Examination of the heart, chest and abdomen was normal. Examination of the central nervous system revealed mild neck stiffness and a positive Kernig's sign.

Investigations: Hb 12.9 g/dl, WBC 9×10^9/l, ESR 45 mm/h, blood sugar 6.4 mmol/l. Urea and electrolytes, liver function tests and chest X-ray were all normal. Lumbar puncture showed 400 white cells per cubic millimetre (70% lymphocytes, 30% neutrophils). CSF protein—1.5 g/l, sugar 2.4 mmol/l, gram and auramine stains of CSF showed no organisms. Culture of CSF was sterile.

In addition to his penicillin, chloramphenicol and sulphadiazine were added to his treatment. The patient remained febrile and unwell. Five days after admission he became drowsy and confused. His neck stiffness and headache worsened and neurological examination showed bilateral brisk reflexes, extensor plantars and impaired upward gaze.

1. What is the most likely diagnosis?
2. What would be the immediate management?

The patient has meningitis with negative bacterial culture which could be due to partially treated bacterial meningitis. The predominance of lymphocytes in the CSF, however, raises the possibility of a viral or tuberculous aetiology, or, more unusually, a fungal or malignant cause. The combination of a lymphocytic pleocytosis and a low CSF sugar should be assumed to be due to **tuberculous meningitis** until proven otherwise. The absence of stainable organisms on direct microscopy does not invalidate the diagnosis, nor would a normal chest X-ray which is present in 25% of patients with tuberculous meningitis. Treatment should begin at once with **triple therapy: rifampicin, isoniazid** and **pyrazinamide. Ethambutol** is sometimes also used. Treatment should continue for 18–24 months.

Subsequent events are suggestive of raised intracranial pressure and mid-brain distortion. In this context, the development of a **communicating hydrocephalus** is the most likely diagnosis because of impaired resorption of CSF due to damage to the arachnoid granulations by meningitis.

Immediate management includes a **CT brain scan** to look for dilated ventricles and possible peri-ventricular lucencies (implying a recent acute rise of intracranial pressure). It will also help to exclude a cerebral abscess, especially if contrast medium is given. Management includes high dose **corticosteroids** (although the use of corticosteroids remains unproven and controversial) and transfer to a neurosurgical centre for consideration of ventricular drainage. The CSF must be examined again in a further attempt to isolate Mycobacteria and exclude other possible causes of aseptic meningitis. The CSF should be examined for malignant cells and fungal and bacterial infections excluded with Indian ink and gram staining respectively. A viral meningo-encephalitis could cause a similar clinical picture and CSF and serum should be sent for viral studies to exclude this retrospectively. The diagnosis of partially treated pyogenic meningitis is often very difficult, but serology may again be helpful. Sarcoidosis and collagen diseases may both cause meningeal involvement, but both are rare and clinical and other laboratory evidence is necessary in making these diagnoses.

The mortality of tuberculous meningitis remains as high as 15–30% in the UK.

Case 91

A 78-year-old lady was admitted for investigation. For the past two months she had been generally unwell, lethargic and anorectic and complaining of generalized muscular pains and arthralgia in shoulders, hips and wrists. Her general practitioner had tried her on an iron/folate combination after vitamin tablets had not improved her symptoms. On the week before admission she had become slightly confused at night with a tendency to fall.

Past medical history included a cholecystectomy 30 years ago and a myocardial infarction six years previously, from which she had made a good recovery. She had been on bendrofluazide 10 mg daily since her myocardial infarction.

On examination she was well orientated, with a temperature of 37.3 °C. Her conjunctivae were pale with two small petechiae on the left. She was not cyanosed or dyspnoeic. Her blood pressure was 160/95 mmHg; pulse 100 beats per minute and regular with a fair volume. The left ventricle was enlarged. The heart sounds were normal with a soft pansystolic murmur at the apex. Her respiratory system was normal, and in the abdomen the spleen tip was just palpable. The central nervous system was normal, with no proximal muscle weakness. General examination showed osteoarthritis of the left knee and Heberden nodes on the fingers. Both temporal arteries were palpable and non-tender.

Investigations showed: Hb 9.8 g/dl, MCV 86 fl, MCHC 30 g/dl, WBC 8.6 × 10⁹/l, platelets 470 × 10⁹/l, ESR 78 mm/h. Urea and electrolytes and liver function tests were normal. Chest X-ray showed left apical calcification and moderate cardiomegaly. Serum B12 and red cell folate were normal. Serum iron was 10 μmol/l. Total iron binding capacity was 36 μmol/l. MSU showed four red cells/high powered field, with no growth.

1. What is the diagnosis?
2. How would you confirm the diagnosis and give six other useful investigations.

This patient demonstrates the non-specific presentation of illness in the elderly. She is anaemic with splenomegaly, red cells in the urine and a vasculitic lesion on the left conjunctiva. In addition, she has the murmur of mitral incompetence and this is strongly suggestive of **infective endocarditis**. The elderly often present with little or no fever and with a long non-specific history. Several other diagnoses should be considered, e.g. polymyalgia rheumatica, tuberculosis and disseminated malignancy. In this case, a renal tumour is a possibility and **renal ultrasound, intravenous urography** and **urine cytology** should be performed.

The anaemia is that of chronic disorder. A myeloproliferative disorder could present in this way and a **blood film** may reveal immature cells. **Bone marrow examination** may show stem cell replacement with tumour, myeloma or fibrosis. This should also be **cultured** for tubercle bacilli and **culture** of **sputum** for *M. Tuberculosis* performed. The diagnosis is made by **blood cultures**, the most common organisms being *Staphylococcus epidermidis* or *Streptococcus viridans*. The haematuria in subacute bacterial endocarditis is multifactorial, but is usually due to immune complex glomerulonephritis and is suggested by a C_3 hypocomplementaemia in the serum.

The most important further investigation, excluding blood cultures, is an **echocardiogram**. This may show valvular vegetations and can assess ventricular and valve function. Transthoracic echocardiography is less sensitive in the detection of small vegetations than transoesophageal echo.

Case 92

A 34-year-old woman presented at the dermatology outpatients after urgent referral from her GP. She had a widespread rash affecting her mucous membranes, arms, palms of her hands and soles of her feet which had started one day previously. Before the rash occurred she had been feeling unwell for several days and had been started on antibiotics for a respiratory tract infection five days before. She had not been abroad and had no history of contact with anyone with a similar disease.

On examination she was ill, pyrexial (38.5°C) and had erythematous macules in different stages of evolution on her palms, arms, soles of her feet and orogenital mucosa. She also had injected eyes and small ulcers on her conjunctivae. Some of the skin lesions had a central blister.

1. What is this condition and give three possible aetiologies?
2. What four investigations would you perform?

This is a typical case of severe **erythema multiforme** or Stevens–Johnson syndrome and she has some lesions with a central blister, typical of the target lesions seen in this condition. The underlying aetiology of this condition is frequently not found, but here a **drug sensitivity** rash is most likely. These are commonly associated with sulphonamides and penicillin antibiotics, which she may well have had. Other important causes of erythema multiformae include **Streptococcal infections** and **viral infections** such as Herpes simplex. Other diagnoses are much less likely. However, with lesions on the palms and soles of the feet, **secondary syphilis** the great mimicker, must be considered. With orogenital ulceration and bullous lesions diseases such as pemphigus and pemphigoid should be considered, though she is young for these and pemphigus has a more protracted course. Pemphigoid and another possibility, bullous dermatitis herpetiformis, are more chronic and have less mucous membrane involvement and fewer systemic symptoms. She does not have any of the other features seen in Beçhet's syndrome. This is unlike chickenpox (polymorphic rash) and the only other possibilities would include septicaemia or systemic lupus erythematosus, or rarely a lymphoma.

Investigation must be aimed initially at finding an aetiological agent. As the lesion is produced by an immune complex, the antigen should be sought looking for Streptococci by **throat swabs** and **blood culture**, and an **ASOT** and sequential **viral studies** should be performed. **Serological tests for syphilis** should also be done. **Secondary infection** should be sought by culturing lesions and collecting blood cultures. If there is any doubt about the diagnosis, **skin biopsy** will confirm the diagnosis and exclude rarer diagnoses such as pemphigus, pemphigoid, dermatitis herpetiformis and lymphomas.

Case 93

A 72-year-old man was brought to casualty by his grandson. While working on the boiler of his houseboat 18 hours previously he suddenly began to feel dizzy and nauseated. The right half of his body tingled and he collapsed, although he did not think that he had lost consciousness. He did not remember many details of the incident. His grandson had found him lying on the floor covered in soot. He was a known hypertensive but had always refused to take medication. He smoked a pipe and drank one bottle of whisky each week.

Examination revealed a well-looking man with equivocal signs of an upper motor neurone lesion affecting the right arm and leg. Examination of the cranial nerves was normal, including funduscopy. Blood pressure was 180/100 mmHg in the left arm and 170/95 mmHg in the right arm. He had several tattoos on his arms. There were no vascular bruits, and the rest of the examination was normal.

Investigations: Hb 16.5 g/dl, WBC 12 × 10⁹/l, platelets 321 × 10⁹/l, sodium 134 mmol/l, potassium 4.8 mmol/l, urea 10.2 mmol/l, creatinine 170 μmol/l, glucose 6.3 mmol/l. Chest X-ray was normal, and ECG showed sinus rhythm with right bundle branch block.

A diagnosis of transient cerebral ischaemia was made, and he was admitted and commenced on aspirin. That evening, the on-call house physican was asked to see him because of a painful swollen right calf. He made a clinical diagnosis of deep venous thrombosis and commenced intravenous heparin. The following morning, the calf was still painful, and both ankles were now swollen. The medical team were surprised to find that blood tests now revealed: sodium 128 mmol/l, potassium 6.8 mmol/l, urea 58 mmol/l, creatinine 1800 μmol/l.

1. What is the diagnosis?
2. Suggest one investigation which would support the diagnosis.
3. Suggest five important aspects of his management.
4. Suggest two alternative diagnoses.

Following a collapse diagnosed as a transient ischaemic attack, this man lay on the floor for 18 hours and subsequently developed a swollen painful calf and acute renal failure. The diagnosis is **rhabdomyolysis** causing acute renal failure due to **myoglobinuria**. The swollen calf represented a compartment syndrome, not a deep venous thrombosis.

Originally described by Bywaters during World War Two as the 'crush syndrome' affecting air-raid victims, the causes of rhabdomyolysis are now known to be numerous. These include prolonged immobility, as in this man's case, polymyositis, heat stroke, prolonged convulsions, carbon monoxide poisoning, heroin abuse and infective causes such as viral necrotizing myositis. Released myoglobin, with a lower molecular weight than haemoglobin, is subject to glomerular filtration and causes acute renal failure both by a direct toxic effect upon the tubules, and by precipitation and obstruction of the tubular system.

Investigations include estimation of blood **creatine phosphokinase** and **aldolase**. These muscle enzymes are greatly elevated in rhabdomyolysis. A specific assay is now available to detect **myoglobin** in blood and in urine.

The management is that of acute renal failure. Careful **fluid balance, dietary protein** and **potassium restriction** and aggressive management of **infection** are vital. **Dialysis** may be indicated, particularly if the patient is anuric. The main indications for dialysis are **fluid overload, symptomatic uraemia** and uncontrollable **hyperkalaemia** and **acidosis**. Most patients with rhabdomyolysis-induced renal failure recover.

A possible alternative diagnosis which may link together both the cerebrovascular event and the acute renal failure is an **aortic dissecting aneurysm**. This could have affected both the cerebral and the renal circulations. However, it is less likely with no chest or back pain following admission. A vasculitis such as **polyarteritis nodosum** may also explain the dual pathology and should be investigated.

Case 94

A 50-year-old previously healthy accountant was brought to casualty with a two day history of progressively more bizarre and aggressive behaviour. On the day of admission she had uncharacteristically begun to shout abuse at her husband and had subsequently become drowsy. When the GP arrived to examine her, she had again become aggressive and abusive. She was taking no medications.

On examination, she was febrile with a temperature of 38.8°C. She was drowsy and opened her eyes in response to loud commands. All her limbs were seen to move spontaneously; her left arm was noted to be twitching continuously. She was moaning incoherently. Her neck was held rigid. There were no other neurological signs.

Investigations: full blood count, urea and electrolytes normal, random glucose 8.4 mmol/l. ECG and chest X-ray were normal. A contrast-enhanced computerized tomograph (CT scan) of the brain showed a low-density, non-enhancing area in the left temporal lobe, which was swollen. An electroencephalogram (EEG) showed recurring complexes over the left temporal lobe. Examination of the cerebrospinal fluid: opening pressure 22 cm CSF, clear and colourless, 45 lymphocytes/mm³, 255 red blood cells/mm³, protein 0.55 g/l, glucose 6.5 mmol/l.

1. What is the most likely diagnosis?
2. Suggest three further investigations.
3. What is the immediate treatment?

This woman presents with confusion and uncharacteristically disturbed, aggressive behaviour. She now has impaired conscious level, meningism, fever and evidence of focal seizure activity. The CT brain scan shows swelling and a low density region in the temporal lobe, and the CSF shows a lymphocytosis with some red cells and a normal CSF to blood glucose ratio. These features are highly suggestive of a diagnosis of **herpes simplex encephalitis**. Other viral causes are possible although less likely. This condition may present in patients who have no previous history of herpes simplex infection, although there may be a history of previous genital or orofacial herpes.

The diagnosis is confirmed by **cerebrospinal fluid viral culture** and by **rising anti-herpes simplex antibody** titres in blood or CSF. Both these diagnostic techniques are helpful in making the diagnosis retrospectively, and hence treatment should be commenced immediately based upon clinical judgement. The **polymerase chain reaction** is being developed as an early diagnostic tool, allowing amplification and measurement of minute quantities of herpes simplex DNA from CSF. This technique is not yet widely available. **Brain biopsy** is rarely carried out in the UK.

Treatment is urgent and is with intravenous **acyclovir**. This antiviral agent with few serious side-effects has transformed the prognosis of herpes simplex encephalitis; however, even with treatment, severe cases with coma are associated with an approximately 20% mortality. In patients who recover there is a significant incidence of profound anterograde amnesia.

Case 95

A 60-year-old boilerhouse operator was admitted from casualty with a 36-hour history of severe constant epigastric pain associated with sweating. The pain gradually eased after diamorphine administration. He had no nausea, vomiting or alteration in bowel habit. He was initially seen by the surgical registrar who did not feel that this pain represented an 'acute abdomen'. In the preceding week he had suffered daily exertional central chest and epigastric tightness. He had no relevant past history and took no medications. He smoked 15 cigarettes daily and drank five pints of beer each week.

On examination he looked comfortable and was afebrile. He was noted to have nicotine-stained fingers. His pulse was 60/min, regular, and blood pressure 120/60 mmHg in both arms. His peripheries were warm and well-perfused. His venous pressure was 12 cm above the sternal angle. His heart sounds were normal and examination of the chest was normal, as was the nervous system. In the abdomen, there was no evidence of peritonism but there was dullness to percussion in the right upper quadrant. He had mild bilateral ankle oedema.

Investigations: Hb 15.0 g/dl, WBC 17.9 × 10^9/l, platelets 239 × 10^9/l, sodium 130 mmol/l, potassium 4.4 mmol/l, urea 9.0 mmol/l, glucose 7.0 mmol/l, amylase normal, liver function tests normal. Erect chest and supine abdominal X-rays were both normal. ECG showed complete heart block with a junctional escape rhythm at a rate of 60/min. There were deep Q-waves with ST segment elevation and T-wave inversion in leads II, III and aVf.

In view of the long history of pain which began to settle he was not given thrombolysis. As his ventricular rate was felt to be adequate, a temporary pacing wire was not inserted. He was given 40 mg frusemide i.v. in view of the raised venous pressure and oedema.

30 minutes later, without further pain, his BP was 60/40 mmHg, pulse 60/min. He was sweating profusely but had no new physical signs. His ECG and chest X-ray were unchanged.

1. What is the most likely diagnosis?
2. Suggest three useful further investigations.
3. Why did he deteriorate?

This man presents with a week of exertional chest and epigastric tightness culminating in a prolonged episode of pain. Examination initially reveals an elevated venous pressure, peripheral oedema and possible hepatomegaly. These features are compatible with 'right heart failure'. It is important to note that there is no evidence initially of 'left heart failure', with an adequate systemic blood pressure and no evidence of pulmonary oedema either clinically or radiographically. The ECG is compatible with acute inferior myocardial infarction with complete heart block but a 'fast' ventricular escape rate. Following diuretic therapy he became hypotensive.

These features are in keeping with **right ventricular myocardial infarction**. This can accompany left ventricular infarction, especially affecting the inferior wall, due to occlusion of the right coronary artery; some postmortem studies have shown that 20% of inferior myocardial infarctions have significant associated right ventricular involvement. Further investigations should include **echocardiography** which in this case showed a hugely dilated right ventricle with poor systolic function, a good left ventricle and normal valves. Although transoesophageal echo may give better views than transthoracic echo, the latter would be performed in the context of acute myocardial infarction. An ECG using **right-sided chest leads** (i.e. RV1-RV6) will show Q-waves and ST segment elevation in the right ventricular leads, especially RV4. **Swan–Ganz catheterization** would allow simultaneous measurement of right heart pressures, pulmonary artery wedge pressure and cardiac output. In this case, the wedge pressure was low and right-sided pressures high.

His deterioration was due to the **administration of diuretic**. This case illustrates the important point that a raised venous pressure and peripheral oedema do not automatically indicate that treatment. On the contrary, the infarcted right ventricle is dependant upon its high preload to maintain cardiac output, and **fluids** in the form of colloid should be given initially to try to improve the situation should the PA wedge pressure be so low as to compromise left ventricular performance. Pulmonary oedema will not form as long as:

$$\text{PA wedge pressure} < 0.57 \times (\text{albumin concentration}) \, \text{mmHg}.$$

If fluids fail, *inotropes* may be necessary. The outcome in right ventricular infarction is often poor, some authorities citing as high as a 40% mortality rate.

Case 96

A 22-year-old Turkish man, studying history at the local university, presented to casualty complaining of lower left pleuritic chest pain. This had started suddenly that morning and gradually worsened. There had been no associated cough or haemoptysis. In addition, he had noticed some tenderness of his right lower leg.

He was normally well, although he had had to drop out of the university hockey team on two occasions during the previous winter due to pain and swelling in firstly his left knee and then his right ankle. The team doctor had evidently attributed these to trauma during preceding games.

He was on no regular medication but took an occasional aspirin for headaches, smoked 5–10 cigarettes per day and did not drink. One month earlier he had returned from visiting his mother in Turkey. His father had died of 'fluid overload' in his early thirties.

On examination, he was febrile with a temperature of 39.2 and had obvious severe pleuritic chest pain with rapid shallow respirations. There was some local chest wall tenderness over the area of pain and breath sounds were diminished. A pleural rub could not be heard. On the skin of his right leg below the knee was a hot tender swollen erythematous area approximately 4 × 7 cm.

Investigations in casualty showed: Hb 14.4 g/dl, WBC 12 × 10⁹/l (N = 70%, L = 26%, M = 2%, E = 2%), ESR 50 mm/h. Urea and electrolytes normal. ECG—sinus tachycardia but otherwise normal. Chest X-ray showed a small left pleural effusion. Urinalysis: protein + + + +, blood negative, glucose negative. Urine microscopy revealed no cells or organisms.

1. What is the diagnosis?
2. What is the likely outcome of the acute attack?
3. What is the long-term prognosis?
4. How would you treat the condition?

This man presents with the typical features of **familial Mediterranean fever**. This is an inherited disease occurring in populations originating on the South and East coasts of the Mediterranean and usually seen elsewhere in Sephardic Jews, and in Arabs.

The disease consists of repeated attacks of fever and painful serositis manifest usually as synovitis, abdominal pain or pleurisy. In some cases, the attacks are associated with an erysipelas-like skin lesion on the lower leg, as in this man. Attacks occur unpredictably and are of sudden onset with fever as a prominent early symptom. Pain and fever generally begin to abate after a few hours and recovery is usually complete in 48 hours although joint effusions may take much longer to resolve, and may occasionally be chronic.

A proportion of patients with familial Mediterranean fever develop amyloidosis and proteinuria can occur either before or at a variable time after the other features of the disease. Renal failure secondary to amyloidosis used to be the usual mode of death, but patients are now treated with dialysis and transplantation.

An effective therapy for the febrile episodes has now been found with patients taking regular **colchicine** which both reduces the frequency and severity of the attacks. Once an attack is established there is little to be done beyond providing pain relief. There is hope that colchicine therapy may hinder the development of amyloidosis.

Despite the typical features other causes for this man's symptoms must be considered. A primary lobar pneumonia is not uncommon in this age group and may initially have no radiological signs. A pleural effusion however would be unlikely without evidence of consolidation. Tuberculosis is a distinct possibility in those from the middle-east but is unlikely to present so acutely. A pulmonary embolism would not cause so high a fever. Systemic lupus erythematosus could cause many of the features but is rare in young men and attacks as acute as this one would be uncommon. Polyarteritis nodosa is unlikely to cause such pronounced proteinuria and the joint symptoms.

Case 97

A 36-year-old Spanish waitress was admitted three days after returning from Madrid, with severe colicky central abdominal pain, radiating to the back. When admitted she passed one loose stool. Her periods were regular. There was no significant past medical history and she was on no medication.

On examination, her temperature was 38.5°C and she was sweating profusely. Her pulse was 120 per minute, regular; blood pressure 160/110 mmHg. There was generalized abdominal tenderness, but no guarding. Rectal examination was normal, and there was no blood or mucus in the stool. Examination of the heart, chest and central nervous system was normal. Vaginal examination was also normal.

Investigations: Hb 12.8 g/dl, WBC 11.0 × 10⁹/l, reticulocytes 1%. Sodium 138 mmol/l, potassium 3.4 mmol/l, urea 3.8 mmol/l. The aspartate transaminase was raised at 48 U/l, but the serum albumin, alkaline phosphatase and bilirubin were normal. Serum amylase was 240 U/l. Stool culture grew no pathogens. Midstream specimen of urine was sterile and contained no cells. Plain abdominal X-ray and chest X-ray were normal. Ward testing of urine (Dipstick) showed urobilinogen + 1, but no bile.

The patient was thought to have cholecystitis, but despite treatment with nasogastric suction, intravenous fluids, analgesia and broad spectrum antibiotics, her condition failed to improve. Over the next 72 hours, her fever continued and she developed increasing abdominal pain.

At laparotomy, the small bowel was rather dilated, but there was no evidence of intestinal obstruction. The gall bladder contained a single small stone, but there was no evidence of acute inflammation. Cholecystectomy was performed and a normal appendix removed. Postoperatively she had further abdominal pain, persistent tachycardia and a prolonged paralytic ileus. She remained febrile. Four days postoperatively her blood pressure dropped from 105/60 mmHg, to 70/40 mmHg, pulse 140 per minute, regular. A chest X-ray was normal and ECG showed a sinus tachycardia. She was thought to have a gram negative septicaemia and was treated with penicillin, gentamicin and metronidazole, as well as intravenous fluids, plasma expanders and hydrocortisone.

Examination of the laparotomy scar showed no evidence of a collection or discharge through the wound. Her intra-abdominal drains showed only a little serous fluid. Her Hb was 12.3 g/dl, WBC 13.0 × 10⁹/l. Sodium 132 mmol/l, potassium 3.6 mmol/l, urea 4.2 mmol/l. Blood sugar 6.3 mmol/l. Blood cultures were sterile on four occasions. A CT scan of the abdomen with contrast enhancement showed no evidence of an intra-abdominal abscess.

1. What is the diagnosis?
2. How would you confirm it?

This lady presented with severe abdominal pain, but no evidence of peritonitis. Following an essentially negative laparotomy, the pain worsened, was associated with a prolonged paralytic ileus and persistent hypotension. Despite adequate treatment of a presumed septicaemia, she remained unwell. Other causes of postoperative deterioration, such as acute myocardial infarction and massive pulmonary embolism were excluded. An intra-abdominal abscess was excluded by CT scanning and perioperative perforation of a viscus was clinically unlikely.

It is in these circumstances that **acute intermittent porphyria** should be considered: the severity of the abdominal pain with an incongruous paucity of physical signs, deterioration following an anaesthetic (barbiturates), and labile blood pressure are all features of this condition. Other modes of presentation include a peripheral polyneuropathy (motor and sensory), and psychiatric disorders including depression and acute psychosis.

The diagnosis rests upon the demonstration of increased **urinary 5-aminolaevulinate (5-ALA)** and **porphobilinogen (PBG)** which are the hallmarks of an acute attack. As the urine may be negative between attacks, measurement of **red blood cell PBG deaminase** and **5-ALA synthetase** activity is very sensitive and may be necessary.

The urine may turn red or red-brown on standing due to oxidation of PBG to porphobilin. A pointer to the diagnosis may also come from the presence of a normal serum bilirubin (although this may be mildly elevated as may urea and transaminases), and the absence of haemolysis, in the presence of a positive reaction of the urine to Ehrlich's reagent. In this classic test, urinary PBG is detected when equal volumes of urine and Ehrlich's aldehyde are mixed; a red colour is positive. Urobilinogen can also produce a red colour, and in the Watson–Schwartz reaction, the red colour due to PBG persists when chloroform is added.

Management is complicated by the exacerbation of many of the symptoms by a wide range of drugs; the most important measure is avoidance of such precipitating causes. Treatment of an acute attack is supportive, with a high carbohydrate intake, as this may reduce porphyrin overproduction indirectly. Intravenous haematin appears to help. Neurological involvement with inadequate respiration and bulbar symptoms may require prolonged periods of ventilation. It may be fatal. The disease is inherited as a Mendelian dominant and the patient's family should be screened. The disorder has been mapped to chromosome 11.

Case 98

A 16-year-old cashier presented to casualty with a two week history of swelling of her ankles. Shortly before the onset of this, she said that she had had an upper respiratory tract infection and sore throat but had recovered uneventfully. She was otherwise well, smoked 20 cigarettes per day and drank an occasional Babycham. She was on no medication.

In her past history she had suffered from the usual childhood diseases and had had her appendix removed two years previously. Her father was a diabetic controlled on insulin and there was no family history of renal disease.

On examination, she looked well, but had rather sunken cheeks. Her mother stated that she had had a normal round face until shortly after an attack of measles at the age of six years. Her blood pressure was 145/80 mmHg and her venous pressure not raised. She had pitting oedema of both ankles to mid-thigh level. Routine urinalysis showed + + + protein and a moderate amount of blood.

Investigations initially showed: Hb 11.7 g/dl, WBC 11.2 × 10⁹/l, ESR 50 mm/h. Her electrolytes were normal and a blood urea 4.0 mmol/l, with serum creatinine 120 μmol/l. Total plasma protein 50 g/l, with albumin 18 g/l. Fasting glucose 5.0 mmol/l. Anti-nuclear factor negative. IVP normal. 24 hour urine protein 12 g (normal < 0.15 g).

1. What is the diagnosis?
2. What complement abnormality would you expect to find?
3. What is the treatment and prognosis?

This girl presents with oedema, hypoproteinaemia and heavy proteinuria, all characteristic of the **nephrotic syndrome**. Hypercholesterolaemia is often present. In addition, she has the characteristic facies of **partial lipodystrophy**. In this condition, there is symmetrical loss of fat from the face with or without disappearance of fat from the arms, chest, abdomen and hips, but with normal distribution of the lower extremities. The aetiology is unknown, but an infective illness is often present at the onset. It is commoner in females and usually presents between 5–15 years of age.

Roughly one-quarter to one-third of patients with partial lipodystrophy have a clinical nephritis and a much larger proportion have complement abnormalities. The characteristic renal lesion is **type 2 mesangiocapillary glomerulonephritis** (MCGN) where histology shows moderately hypercellular glomeruli with thickened capillary loops. There is mesangial cell proliferation and electron microscopy shows dense linear intramembranous deposits which stain positive for C3.

The complement abnormality seen is a **low serum C3 concentration**, with normal levels of the earlier components of the classical pathway, CIq, C4 and C2. This suggests that C3 is activated via the alternative pathway and the C3 **nephritic factor** has been found in the serum of these patients.

The course of type 2 MCGN is of continuing disease with slow decline into renal failure. There is no good evidence that steroids or immunosuppressants modify the course.

Symptomatic treatment of the nephrotic syndrome with diuretics may be necessary and supporting stockings are often helpful. Hypertension and urinary tract infections should be watched for and treated. When renal failure intervenes, she will require treatment with dialysis and possible transplantation.

Case 99

A 64-year-old man presented to casualty with a three-hour history of severe central chest pain and dyspnoea. He had no relevant previous history and smoked 10 cigarettes daily.

Examination was normal.

Investigations: full blood count, urea and electrolytes and glucose normal. Chest X-ray normal. ECG showed sinus rhythm with 2 mm ST segment elevation in leads V1–V3.

A diagnosis of acute myocardial infarction was made. He was admitted to the coronary care unit and given analgesia, antiemetics, oxygen, aspirin, intravenous thrombolysis and a heparin infusion. His pain settled and he suffered no rhythm disturbance or heart failure.

Three days after admission he developed a purpuric eruption and nail fold infarcts on both feet. The rest of the examination was normal.

1. Suggest three possible reasons for this development.
2. Suggest four useful further investigations.

This man has had an acute myocardial infarction and has received thrombolytic therapy and heparin. He has subsequently developed a vasculitic process affecting his feet.

He may have a **vasculitis** relating to **streptokinase** therapy; this occurs particularly in those who have received previous streptokinase therapy, although it can occur on the first exposure in those who have had previous Streptococcal infection. It is an immune-complex phenomenon and **anti-streptokinase antibodies** can be measured. **Complement levels, ESR, C-reactive protein** and **circulating immune complexes** should be checked. Renal impairment may occur as in other vasculitides and **renal function tests** should be repeated.

Treatment with intravenous heparin, especially if prolonged, can lead to bone marrow suppression and cause **heparin-induced thrombocytopenic syndrome** (**HITS**). This may cause purpura although is less likely to cause nail fold infarcts. A **platelet** count should be repeated.

The features in the legs may be **embolic**. **Mural thrombus** may have developed within the infarcted left ventricle and **echocardiography** should be carried out; transthoracic echo is less sensitive than transoseophageal echo but the latter should not be carried out so soon after an acute myocardial infarction. In view of the distribution of the lesions, the source of the emboli may be in the **aorta** above the bifurcation. There are case reports of thrombus and cholesterol embolization from atheromatous abdominal aortas following thromblytic therapy.

Finally, the acute myocardial infarction may have been due not to coronary atheroma but as part of a generalized vasculitis such as **polyarteritis nodosum**. Although this is less likely, a full **vasculitis screen** should be completed, to include **anti-neutrophil cytoplasmic antibody** (ANCA), which has been associated with microscopic polyarteritis and Wegener's, **anti-nuclear factor** and an **eosinophil** count.

Case 100

A 46-year-old man presented in casualty complaining of the sudden onset of left loin pain radiating to his left groin. He stated that he had had similar previous attacks of pain, usually left-sided but occasionally on the right. He had been told he suffered from renal stones and had been hospitalized several times in Ireland, the last time six months previously. In his past history he had also had an operation for an ulcer and operations for adhesions, all in Ireland. He was a labourer, unmarried and had come to England three months ago. He lived in a bedsit and denied any drugs or medications.

On examination he was writhing in agony and was afebrile. Abdominal examination showed four laparotomy scars and he was slightly tender in the left loin. There were what appeared to be venepuncture marks on the right arm.

Initial investigations: Hb 14.5 g/dl, WBC 7.4 × 109/l, ESR 4 mm/h, urea and electrolytes normal. Chest X-ray and abdominal X-ray were both normal. Urinalysis–blood + +.

A diagnosis of left renal colic was made, he was given a dose of pethidine and admitted under the urologists where a subsequent MSU was sterile and an IVP was normal. Daily urinalysis confirmed persistent haematuria.

He complained of no further loin pain but two days later developed tight central chest pain radiating to the left arm. On examination, he was not sweating or dyspnoeic, but seemed in severe pain. Pulse 72/minute and regular, blood pressure 110/70 mmHg, venous pressure not raised, heart sounds normal, chest clinically clear. He was given diamorphine and transferred to the coronary unit and kept under bedrest and close observation. His chest X-ray was repeated and was unchanged and serial ECGs showed an old inferior myocardial infarction but did not change. His cardiac enzymes did not become raised and whilst on the coronary unit his haematuria was noted to have disappeared.

1. What is the diagnosis?
2. What is the treatment and prognosis?

This man gives two classical clinical histories, firstly of renal colic, and secondly of ischaemic heart disease, neither of which is substantiated on investigation. In addition, his past medical history is made difficult to confirm, he has multiple laparotomy scars and has possibly had a recent hospital admission, as evidenced by venepuncture marks. All these make it likely that he is suffering from **Munchausen's syndrome**. In addition, his haematuria, readily faked when on a general ward, disappeared when he was kept under close observation.

Munchausen's syndrome is applied to patients who have made hospital admission a way of life. They often present with dramatic symptoms and can go to elaborate lengths to feign their disease; many with chest pain often have abnormal ECGs, as with this man. The symptomatology is often wide and when one group of symptoms is in danger of being discovered a fake, they may change to a second group. They often have evidence of multiple previous operations, usually laparotomy scars or burr holes. The past medical history they give may be elaborate and is usually extremely difficult to substantiate. This problem is increased by the fact that they often use differing names at their admissions.

The syndrome is named after a fanciful character of fiction, Baron Munchausen, who was himself based on an 18th century Hanoverian army officer of the same name. Both these characters were renowed for exaggerated and extraordinary stories.

Most Munchausen patients take their own discharge as soon as discovery is imminent. Hence, evaluation of the psychopathology is difficult, let alone the fact that they are known to be individuals who deliberately lie to mislead. It is seldom justifiable to detain such patients compulsively and with their elusive nature no treatment can usually be offered. This is perhaps just as well as no effective treatment is known and failure has been reported with hypnosis, ECT and leucotomy. The patient's elusiveness makes long-term outcome uncertain.

Their multiple hospital admissions distinguish them from simple **malingerers** and the short non-continuing nature of this man's pain together with the absence of any withdrawal symptoms, make it unlikely that he is a **drug addict** wanting more of his drug.

If possible, it is helpful to obtain a photograph of the patient for any subsequent identification.

Index to Diagnoses and Differential Diagnoses

Numbers refer to pages